The Executive Years of the NHS

The England Account 1985–2003

Brian Edwards

Emeritus Professor of Health Care Development
School of Health and Related Research
University of Sheffield

and

Margaret Fall

Research Fellow
School of Health and Related Research
University of Sheffield

Foreword by

Sir Denis Pereira Gray

Chairman of the Trustees
The Nuffield Trust

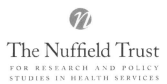

The Nuffield Trust

FOR RESEARCH AND POLICY
STUDIES IN HEALTH SERVICES

Radcliffe Publishing

Oxford • Seattle

Radcliffe Publishing Ltd
18 Marcham Road
Abingdon
Oxon OX14 1AA
United Kingdom

www.radcliffe-oxford.com
Electronic catalogue and worldwide online ordering facility.

British Library Cataloguing in Publication Data

A catalogue record for this book is available from the British Library.

ISBN 1 85775 759 9

Typeset by Anne Joshua & Associates, Oxford
Printed and bound by TJ International Ltd, Padstow, Cornwall

Contents

Foreword

The British National Health Service when it was established in 1948 was the most radical and comprehensive health system in the world. It has since become one of the largest employers in Europe and is now receiving the largest proportional increase in government funding of any public service since the Second World War. It is therefore natural that it is being studied increasingly by historians, by academics in social policy and political science, and by the health professions involved.

The Nuffield Trust had long sought to illuminate public policy on health and healthcare. It hopes that this new contribution, from a managerial perspective, will complement another book which the Trust is soon to publish, called *The Nation's Doctor* on the office of the Chief Medical Officer.[1]

Around the middle of the 1980s, a major revolution occurred which can be summarised as the rise of management. Until then, much of health policy in Britain had, in effect, been initiated by the health professions, especially doctors and nurses. The stimulus for this change was the Griffiths Report (1983)[2] commissioned by Mrs Thatcher, and the revolution it unleashed has not yet run its course.

The period since 1983 is therefore of special importance and Brian Edwards and Margaret Fall are well placed to describe and analyse it. Professor Edwards was formerly the Regional General Manager in the Midlands, the largest NHS region in England, at a time when the NHS regional health authorities were powerful forces in the land and a significant instrument in devolved decision taking.

This book charts the frenetic change in organisational arrangements which the NHS has experienced and discusses the numerous policy initiatives introduced by governments of different political persuasions, including the abolition of the regional health authorities.

Professor Edwards is well placed both from his own personal experience and also by virtue of the opportunities he had to see central policy papers and meet many of the central personalities. He had a ring side seat for many of the changes in the NHS. This valuable history of the evolving NHS, co-written by Dr Margaret Fall of Sheffield University, will contribute to the current policy debate on attitudes to management and public service.

Sir Denis Pereira Gray
Chairman of the Trustees
The Nuffield Trust
July 2005

References

1 Sheard S and Donaldson L (2006) *The Nation's Doctor: the role of the Chief Medical Officer 1855–1998.* Radcliffe Publishing, Oxford and Seattle. Co-published with The Nuffield Trust.
2 Griffiths R (1983) *Management Inquiry.* HMSO, London.

About the authors

Professor Brian Edwards
Emeritus Professor of Health Care Development
School of Health and Related Research
University of Sheffield

Margaret Fall
Research Fellow
School of Health and Related Research
University of Sheffield

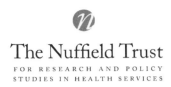

The Nuffield Trust
FOR RESEARCH AND POLICY
STUDIES IN HEALTH SERVICES

The Nuffield Trust is one of the leading independent health policy charitable trusts in the UK. It was established as the Nuffield Provincial Hospitals Trust in 1940 by Viscount Nuffield (William Morris), the founder of Morris Motors. In 1998 the Trustees agreed that the official name of the trust should more fully reflect the Trust's purposes and, in consultation with the Charity Commission, adopted the name The Nuffield Trust for Research and Policy Studies in Health Services, retaining 'The Nuffield Trust' as its working name.

The Nuffield Trust's mission is to promote independent analysis and informed debate on UK healthcare policy. The Nuffield Trust's purpose is to communicate evidence and encourage an exchange around developed or developing knowledge in order to illuminate recognised and emerging issues.

It achieves this through its principal activities:

- Bringing together a wide national and international network of people involved in UK healthcare through a series of meetings, workshops and seminars.
- Commissioning research through its publications and grants programme to inform policy debate.
- Encouraging interdisciplinary exchange between clinicians, leglislators, academics, healthcare professionals and management, policy makers, industrialists and consumer groups.
- Supporting evidence-based health policy and practice.
- Sharing its knowledge in the home countries and internationally through partnerships and alliances.

To find out more please refer to our website or contact:

The Nuffield Trust
59 New Cavendish St
London
W1G 7LP
Website: www.nuffieldtrust.org.uk
Email: mail@nuffieldtrust.org.uk
Tel: +44 (0)20 7631 8458
Fax: +44 (0)20 7631 8451

Charity number: 209201

Acknowledgements

Whenever one embarks on a historical review one builds on the work of others. We have drawn on many sources, but we found three authors in particular of exceptional value. We recommend their work to our readers:

- Ham C (1999) *Health Policy in Britain* (4e). Palgrave Publications, Basingstoke.
- Klein R (2001) *The New Politics of the NHS* (4e). Pearson, Harlow.
- Timmins N (2001) *The Five Giants*. HarperCollins, London.

We are grateful to Members of Parliament, civil servants and NHS staff, both past and present, for their help, including those who agreed to be interviewed about their association with the National Health Service. Our thanks also to our colleagues at the Sheffield University School of Health and Related Research (ScHARR) for their support and comments as our story unfurled, and to Louise Hall and Deborah Owen for their help.

We are extremely grateful for the courtesy and professionalism afforded to us by the staff at the Department of Health file store in Nelson, Lancashire.

List of abbreviations

AGM	Area General Manager
AHA	area health authority
BMA	British Medical Association
CBI	Confederation of British Industry
CHAE	Central Health Authority for England
CHC	Community Health Council
CHI	Commission for Health Improvement
CIP	Cost Improvement Programme
CMO	Chief Medical Officer
CNO	Chief Nursing Officer
DGM	District General Manager
DHA	district health authority
DHSS	Department of Health and Social Security
DMU	district-managed unit
DoH	Department of Health
FHSA	family health services authority
FPC	Family Practitioner Committee
FPS	Family Practitioner Services
GDP	gross domestic product
GMC	General Medical Council
HAZ	Health Action Zone
HPSS	Health and Personal Social Services
HSSB	Health Service Supervisory Board
ITU	intensive-therapy unit
LA	local authority
NAHAT	National Association of Health Authorities and Trusts
NHS	National Health Service
NICE	National Institute for Clinical Excellence
NSF	National Service Framework
PAC	Public Accounts Committee
PCG	primary care group
PCT	primary care trust
PESC	Public Expenditure Survey Committee
PFI	Private Finance Initiative
PLA	Port of London Authority
PPS	Parliamentary Private Secretary
RAWP	Resources Allocation Working Party
RCN	Royal College of Nursing
RGM	Regional General Manager
RHA	regional health authority
RISP	Regional Information Systems Development Plan
SHA	special health authority
TUC	Trades Union Congress

Office holders during the period 1970–2003

Members of Parliament, senior civil servants and NHS staff holding office during the period covered by the Executive years[1]

Date of appointment	Prime Minister
19 June 1970	Edward Heath
04 March 1974	Harold Wilson
05 April 1976	James Callaghan
04 May 1979	Margaret Thatcher
28 November 1990	John Major
02 May 1997	Tony Blair

Date of appointment	Chief Executive
1985–1988	Victor Paige
1986–1989	Len Peach
1989–1994	Duncan Nichol
1994–2000	Alan Langlands
2000	Nigel Crisp

Date of appointment	Chief Medical Officer
1960–1973	George Godber
1973–1983	Henry Yellowlees
1984–1991	Donald Acheson
1991–1998	Kenneth Calman
1998	Liam Donaldson

Date of appointment	Permanent Secretary
1975–1981	Patrick Nairne
1981–1988	Kenneth Stowe
1988–1991	Christopher France
1991–1997	Graham Hart
1997–2000	Chris Kelly
2000	Nigel Crisp

Ministerial Membership of Department of Health and Social Security/Department of Health

Date of appointment	Secretary of State	Party
June 1970	Keith Joseph	Conservative
March 1974	Barbara Castle	Labour
April 1976	David Ennals	Labour
May 1979	Patrick Jenkin	Conservative
September 1981	Norman Fowler	Conservative
June 1987	John Moore	Conservative
July 1988	Kenneth Clarke	Conservative
November 1990	William Waldegrave	Conservative
April 1992	Virginia Bottomley	Conservative
July 1995	Stephen Dorrell	Conservative
May 1997	Frank Dobson	Labour
October 1999	Alan Milburn	Labour
June 2003	John Reid	Labour
May 2005	Patricia Hewitt	Labour

Date of appointment	Minister of State	Party
1970–1974	Lord Aberdare	Conservative
1974	Brian O'Malley	Conservative
1974–1976	David Owen	Labour
1976–1979	Stan Orme	Labour
1976–1979	Roland Moyle	Conservative
1979–1982	Gerald Vaughan	Conservative
1979–1981	Reginald Prentice	Conservative
1981–1982	Hugh Rossie	Conservative
1982–1985	Kenneth Clarke	Conservative
1983–1984	Rhodes Boyson	Conservative
1984–1988	Tony Newton	Conservative
1985–1986	Barney Hayhoe	Conservative
1986–1987	John Major	Conservative
1987–1994	Nicholas Scott	Conservative
1988–1989	David Mellor	Conservative
1989–1992	Virginia Bottomley	Conservative
1992–1994	Brian Mawhinney	Conservative
1994–1997	Gerald Malone	Conservative
1997–1999	Tessa Jowell	Labour
1997–1999	Alan Milburn	Labour
1997–1998	Baroness Jay	Labour
1999–2001	John Denham	Labour
1999–2005	John Hutton	Labour
2001–2003	Jacqui Smith	Labour
2003	Rosie Winterton	Labour
2005	Lord Warner	Labour
2005	Jane Kennedy	Labour

Introduction

The effective management of public services has been close to the centre of political debate in the UK for the last 50 years. Modern history is littered with the wreckage of one attempt or another to reform them and make them perform better. For many years there was clear political water between those on the left, who insisted on public ownership and management, and those on the right, who argued that such services would be provided more efficiently by the private sector. In the last ten years the gap has narrowed with ideas about separating out those who pay for and commission such services and those who actually provide them. All the main parties remain committed to a state-funded National Health Service (NHS), but ideas about separating the providers of service and particularly the hospital sector from government and giving them freedom to operate more like commercial undertakings are now common. Foundation trusts, the latest Labour Party policy plan, have an uncanny similarity to ideas that were considered during the Thatcher review of the NHS but rejected at the time as being too radical.

Government and ministers have, over the last 30 years, oscillated between the micro-management of the NHS from the centre, and standing back from the detail and adopting a more strategic role. Whitehall itself has changed a lot in recent years as ministers have attempted to reduce its role in the detailed provision of services and strengthen its grip on policy development. The creation of Next Steps Agencies was one of the principal policy planks in this process. These organisations, staffed by civil servants, are accountable to ministers but have clear financial and service targets and day-to-day operational freedom. The most obvious examples are the Benefits Agency, the Passport Office, the Meteorological Office and the Driver and Vehicle Licensing Agency.

The NHS in England took a rather different path. It was judged as too big and too sensitive to be turned into a Next Steps Agency. Ideas about a separate NHS Corporation arose on a number of occasions, but were always rejected. Instead the NHS was run from Whitehall with an influx of experienced professionals from outside the civil service serving on an Executive Board. The first Board met in 1985 under the chairmanship of Victor Paige. The last one met in 2001 when the Executive was disbanded. In this book we chart the progression of these Executive Boards in their various guises and the five managers who were appointed to lead them. We have done so against a general history of the NHS during the period, which provides the backcloth and the setting for two major questions. The first is about how government should manage public services and health in particular, and the second is whether the constitutional principle of parliamentary accountability will always demand that a minister be in charge.

As Sir Kenneth Stowe, one of the great mandarins, put it:

> Beginning with Victor Paige and ending with Nigel Crisp, we have been up hill and down dale trying to sort out this division of responsibilities between ministers and permanent secretaries and

something called the Management Board which has outsiders on it. In fact they are outsiders exercising the minister's powers only for as long as he says 'you can have my powers to play with'.[2]

Our telling of the history is selective. In order to explore the big picture we have left out the detail that makes up the true picture of a huge and complex social enterprise. We shall concentrate on England, although the development path in the other parts of the UK was very similar during this period of time.

Chapter 1

Timeline[3]

1968

- Kenneth Robinson's Green Paper[4] on NHS reorganisation in England and Wales was published with a similar paper in December in Scotland. Both proposed the replacement of the tripartite division of health services with area boards (40–50 for England and Wales), combining the responsibilities of Regional Hospital Boards, Hospital Management Committees, local authority personal health services and Executive Councils.
- The Ministries of Health and Social Security were amalgamated to form the Department of Health and Social Security (DHSS). Richard Crossman became the first Secretary of State for Social Services. Health regained its Cabinet seat.

1969

- The Redcliffe Maud Commission on Local Government[5] reported, recommending three Metropolitan Authorities containing 20 Metropolitan District Authorities outside London and 58 Unitary Authorities in the rest of England. They also felt that local authorities should take over responsibility for the NHS.
- The Hospital Advisory Service was established following a series of scandals about the ill-treatment of patients in long-stay hospitals. Geoffrey Howe led an inquiry into care at Ely Hospital in Wales.

1970

- Richard Crossman's Green Paper[6] on NHS reorganisation was published. It amended Robinson's 1968 proposals by doubling the number of area boards to fit in with local government arrangements, it reintroduced the idea of regional planning boards and it suggested, within the larger area boards, local 'district' committees to involve the community and health service workers in running the NHS. However, the chain of command was to run from the minister direct to area boards, with regions having an advisory role only.
- The Conservatives won the General Election. Keith Joseph replaced Richard Crossman as Secretary of State for Social Services.

1971

- The *Harvard Davies Report on the Organisation of GP Group Practice*[7] was published.
- The White Paper *Better Services for the Mentally Handicapped*[8] was published.

1972

- The *Report of the Committee of Inquiry into Whittington Hospital,*[9] arising out of allegations of ill-treatment of patients and theft, was published.
- Keith Joseph's White Paper *National Health Service Reorganisation: England*[10] was published proposing 14 regional health authorities (RHAs) in a direct management line between the Secretary of State and area health authorities (AHAs), no district committees but a Community Health Council (CHC) in each district, Joint Consultative Committees with local authorities, and specialists in community medicine. A similar document was published for Wales.
- *Management Arrangements for the Reorganised National Health Service* (the Grey Book)[11] was published. A similar document was published in September for Wales.

1973

- A report was published by the Working Party on Collaboration between the NHS and Local Government.[12]
- The post of Health Service Commissioner was established, and Sir Alan Marre was appointed.
- On 5 July the National Health Service Reorganisation Act was given the Royal Assent on the twenty-fifth anniversary of the establishment of the NHS.

1974

- The General Election in February gave no party a clear majority. Prime Minister Edward Heath resigned. Harold Wilson became Prime Minister and Barbara Castle was appointed as Secretary of State for Social Services in the resulting Labour Government. Dr David Owen became Minister of Health.
- NHS Reforms on 1 April created 14 Regions and 90 Area Health Boards managing 206 District Management Teams. Family Practitioner Committees (FPCs) were coterminous with and set up by area health authorities. Teams of managers were introduced at district, area and regional level.
- Sir Henry Yellowlees was appointed Chief Medical Officer (CMO) at the Department of Health and Social Security.
- Barbara Castle's consultative document *Democracy in the National Health Service*[13] was published, and resulted in the inclusion of local government representatives on regional health authorities, an increase in their number on area health authorities, and powers for community health councils regarding the approval of hospital closures.
- In the second General Election in October, Labour won with a working majority of three.

1975

- Harold Wilson announced that the Royal Commission on the NHS would be established and chaired by Sir Alec Merrison.

1976

- James Callaghan became Prime Minister in April. David Ennals replaced Barbara Castle as Secretary of State for Social Services.
- The *Regional Chairmen's Inquiry into the Working of the DHSS in Relation to Regional Health Authorities*[14] was published (convened by Dr David Owen, Minister of Health). It recommended a strengthened role for regions and a 'thinned out' Department of Health.
- The Health Services Board was created to phase out private beds in the NHS.
- Sir Patrick Nairne became Permanent Secretary at the DHSS.
- The Resource Allocation Working Party (RAWP) Report, *Sharing Resources for Health in England*,[15] was published.

1977

- The National Health Service Act became law. It largely consolidated previous legislation, but also gave the Government the power to set up special health authorities (SHAs).
- In the Hounslow Raid, health officials 'raided' the Hounslow hospital to remove 21 elderly patients to the Middlesex Hospital to end a 'work-in' by nurses aimed at averting the closure of the ward.

1978

- Declaration of Alma Ata; the World Health Organization produced 'Health for All'.[367]
- In the late 1980s a period of sustained industrial unrest began in Britain, which became known as the 'winter of discontent'. The NHS faced another strong pay campaign from ancillary workers.

1979

- The Conservatives won the General Election in May. Margaret Thatcher became Prime Minister and Patrick Jenkin became Secretary of State for Social Services.
- The *Royal Commission on the NHS*[16] reported that the NHS was 'not in need of major surgery'. The Government later published its own plans for further health service reorganisation.
- Crown Commissioners were contemplated for Lambeth, Southwark and Lewisham (Teaching) Area Health Authorities in the light of their unresolved financial position.
- The Clegg Report, *Pay Comparability*,[17] was published.
- *Patients First*[18] was published by the DHSS in response to the Royal Commission:
  - strengthening management at local level
  - removing the area tier and establishing district health authorities (DHAs)
  - simplifying professional advisory machinery
  - simplifying the planning system.

1980

- The Government reluctantly published the Black Report, *Inequalities in Health*,[19] on poverty and ill health.
- The DHSS published the Nodder Report, *Organisational and Management Problems of Mental Illness Hospitals*.[20]
- The Employment Act banned secondary picketing.
- The Health Services Act:
  - dissolved the Central Health Services Council (the Minister's advisory body)
  - dissolved the Health Services Board, which had been established to phase out private beds
  - disbanded the AHAs and created 192 DHAs in their place.
- *Hospital Services: Future Pattern of Hospital Provision in England*[21] was published, which proposed that District General Hospitals (DGHs) should not exceed 600 beds, and that smaller hospitals should be retained where possible.

1981

- Cost Improvement Programmes were introduced in April.
- *The Harding Report*[22] on Primary Healthcare Teams was published in May.
- Kenneth Stowe became Permanent Secretary to the DHSS in June.
- In September, Norman Fowler became Secretary of State, with Gerald Vaughan, and later Kenneth Clarke, as Minister of Health.

1982

- In January, Norman Fowler announced the creation of annual review meetings with ministers, RHA chairmen and regional officers following pressure from the Public Accounts Committee to strengthen NHS accountability to Parliament. He also announced that performance indicators would be developed.
- In March the health unions started a campaign for a 12% pay rise with a series of one-day strikes. The armed forces were put on standby to cover gaps in emergency services.
- On 1 April the NHS was reorganised again (from the 1979 White Paper and 1980 Health Services Act):
  - the area tier was abolished
  - district health authorities took over as the main operational authorities
  - the 'unit' was established as the local management tier
  - planning procedures were pruned.
- The DHSS announced the extension of Rayner Efficiency Scrutinies into the NHS.
- A review of NHS staffing, which was to lead to the Griffiths Report, was announced at the Conservative Party Conference in September.
- The Körner Report of the Steering Group on Health Services[23] was published in November.

1983

- In January the DHSS announced central control of NHS manpower numbers.
- The Conservatives won a landslide victory in June, and Margaret Thatcher returned as Prime Minister. Norman Fowler stayed on as Secretary of State for Health and Social Security.
- The UK Central Council for Nursing, Midwifery and Health Visiting (UKCC) was established under powers contained in the 1979 Nurses Act.
- Health authorities were instructed by the DHSS to introduce competitive tendering.
- The first set of performance indicators was published.
- The Griffiths Report[24] was published in October, recommending the following:
  - establishment at the centre of a Supervisory Board and an NHS Management Board
  - appointment of a national Director of Personnel
  - regional and district chairmen to extend the accountability review process through to unit level
  - identification of individual general managers for each unit of management
  - introduction of management budgeting relating workload and service objectives to the available financial and manpower resources, and involving clinicians in this.
- Plans to abolish the Greater London Council were announced.
- The Ceri Davies Report[25] on use of NHS land was published.
- The healthcare staff pay dispute was settled.
- The Supervisory Board met for the first time in December and was chaired by Norman Fowler.

1984

- The consultation period on the Griffiths Report ended in January, and the DHSS published the circular on implementation in June.
- *The Report of the NHS Management Inquiry: Implications for the Organisation of the Department*[26] was prepared by Hart and colleagues and was circulated within the DHSS.
- A pay review body for nurses was established.
- An Interim Management Board was set up under the chairmanship of Dr John Evans.
- Headhunters were appointed in March for the post of Chief Executive in the NHS.
- The first abortive interviews were held in September.
- By July, Regional General Managers began to be appointed.
- A salmonella outbreak occurred at Stanley Royd Hospital, Wakefield.
- In October a bomb exploded at the Conservative Party Conference in Brighton.
- A limited drug list was announced, designed to reduce NHS drug expenditure and encourage generic prescribing.
- Optician monopoly of the sale of spectacles ended.
- British Telecom was privatised.
- Donald Acheson took over from Sir Henry Yellowlees as CMO.

Roots of the Griffiths Inquiry

The ideas that led to the appointment of Victor Paige as Chairman of the NHS Management Board for England in January 1985 had their roots in the industrial disputes in the earlier years of the decade, and in two failed attempts to improve the organisation of the NHS by changes to its structure. The 1974 reforms had been designed to bring the statutory family of the NHS, which at this stage encompassed Hospital Management Committees, Executive Councils (which ran Family Practitioner Services) and community services managed by local authorities, together in pursuit of more integrated management and care. These reforms might have worked had they not been accompanied by a novel but ultimately flawed approach to management, which was imposed by the centre.

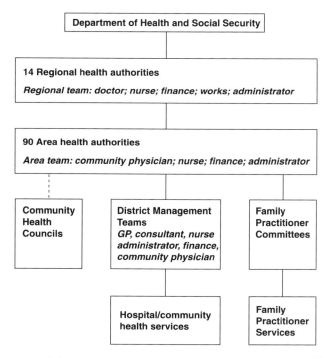

Figure 1.1 Structure of the NHS in England during the period 1974–82.[27]

Every area health authority had a team of officers which handled policy development on its behalf, and a variable number of locality-based district management teams that were responsible to them (but not through the area team) for the day-to-day management of services on the ground. Every detail of the structure and how it would work had been defined by the Department of Health and Social Security in what came to be known as the Grey Book.[11]

Each management team was multi-disciplinary and was required to work on a consensus basis. Every team member had to agree before a decision could be reached. At its best it was a brilliant way of managing a complex multi-professional organisation, and at its worst it was a disaster. In some authorities the officers at area level meddled in day-to-day matters and the district teams fought to secure a role in policy discussions, especially when they impacted on their locality. It was a good example of how difficult it is to separate out policy and day-to-day management. There was tension both within teams and between teams. One of the worst examples was Solihull, where the management team was in perpetual crisis. The team members simply could not talk to each other without quarrelling. An inquiry was ordered which involved a young barrister, Kenneth Clarke, who was later to be the Secretary of State. It was not a good foundation from which to respect health service management.

Kenneth Clarke, Secretary of State, July 1988–90

Kenneth Clarke was born on 2 July 1940 in Nottinghamshire, where his father had been a miner and an electrician but now repaired watches and ran a cinema in Eastwood.

From the local school Clarke won a scholarship to Nottingham High School, where his passions were trainspotting and football. He went up to Gonville and Caius College, Cambridge and became President of the Union. He was recruited by Norman Fowler to the Cambridge Union Conservative Association, where he mixed with John Gummer, Norman Lamont, Leon Brittan and Michael Howard, all of whom were to become leading members of the Tory Party.

He was called to the Bar in 1963 and worked as a barrister before becoming MP for Rushcliffe in Nottingham in 1970. In Parliament he worked with Norman Fowler in the Department of Industry and Transport. From 1982 to 1985 Clarke was Minister of Health. In 1985 he entered the Cabinet as Paymaster General and Minister for Employment. From 1988 to 1990 he was Secretary of State for Health. He launched the internal market in the NHS in the wake of the Thatcher Review, and played a major role in determining the detail of that reform. He moved on before it became operational to become Secretary of State for Education and Science (1990–1992), Home Secretary (1992–1993) and Chancellor of the Exchequer (1993–1997).

Complaints about the bureaucratic nature of the 1974 reforms had made it necessary to set up a Royal Commission in 1975, some 18 months after the reforms had been introduced. This reported in 1979 that the NHS 'was not suffering from a mortal disease susceptible only to heroic surgery.'[16] What was needed, the Royal Commission argued, was to keep on with the long slog of improving performance.

The Government did not agree, and in 1982 the area tier was removed by the then Secretary of State, Norman Fowler. District health authorities took over the planning and management of the hospital and community health services in their locality. The family health services (the independent contractors in primary care, such as GPs) were now to be managed separately by new bodies called family health services authorities (FHSAs). These would report directly to the Department of Health.

Integrated service management, which was the policy driver of the 1974 reforms, no longer seemed important, perhaps because the family health services had determinedly retained their separateness from the hospital world inside the supposedly integrated 1974 structures. It was an example of how inadequate structural solutions are for complex service delivery problems.

Norman Fowler, Secretary of State, 1981–87

Norman Fowler was born in 1938 in Chelmsford, where he went to grammar school. After national service with the Essex Regiment, he went to Cambridge University in 1958 to read law. By 1960 he was Chairman of the Cambridge University Conservative Association. Also at Cambridge at the same time were John Gummer (President of the Union), Leon Brittan, Kenneth Clarke, Michael Howard, John Nott and Norman Lamont.

Fowler began work as a reporter for *The Times* newspaper in 1961, and later became the first Home Office Correspondent for *The Times*.

In June 1970 he stood for Parliament and was elected as MP for South Nottingham and later Sutton Coldfield. A series of opposition front-bench appointments followed. He became Minister of Transport in 1979 and chose Ken Clarke as his deputy in 1980. Around this time he made the remark 'Civil servants tell you the case which will be made out against your policies and they give you their views, but in the end it is the Minister who decides'.

In September 1981 Margaret Thatcher appointed Fowler as Secretary of State for Health and Social Services and said at the party conference 'The Health Service is safe with us'. Fowler commissioned the Griffiths Management Enquiry. After the 1987 General Election, he moved to the Department of Employment and John Moore took over at the DHSS.

In 1990, at the age of 51 years, Fowler resigned so that he would be able to spend more time with his family, although he returned to active politics in 1992 as Chairman of the Conservative Party.

Despite these changes, Fowler was still not convinced that the organisation was right, particularly at the DHSS. He observed a clear distinction between the various parts of his huge empire. 'As far as Health was concerned we didn't have management skills within the Department. The civil servants were advisers to me. By contrast, Social Security was directly managed; they managed the Benefit Shops and the rest, and were responsible for it.'[29]

In 1982, the health trade unions asked for a uniform flat-rate settlement of 12% for all NHS employees. The Government decided to resist the claim and if necessary face up to industrial action. A figure of 12% was simply too inflationary. According to Sir Kenneth Stowe, the Permanent Secretary, it was also 'essential for good management that the concept of a uniform flat-rate increase for all, irrespective of demand, skill, performance and ability to pay, be overturned.'[2]

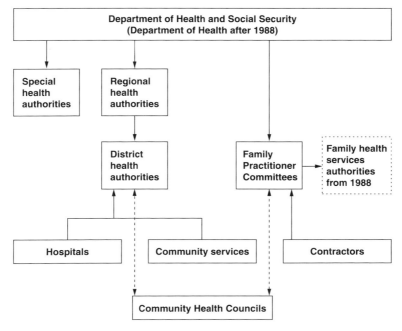

Figure 1.2 Structure of the NHS in England during the period 1982–91.[27, 28]

   The dispute began in March 1982 with a selective series of one-day stoppages. For many this was like going back to the bad old days of the winter of discontent in 1978–79, which had badly bruised both the DHSS and the Trades Union Congress (TUC). By the summer of 1982, services were seriously disrupted and in some places emergency services were jeopardised. On 22 September thousands of people marched through London in what *The Times* called 'the biggest revolt of the decade'. Troops were put on one-hour standby to cover any gaps in the ambulance service in the capital.

Kenneth Stowe, Permanent Secretary, 1981–87

Kenneth Stowe was educated at the County High School, Dagenham, and at Oxford University, where he gained a degree in modern history. He worked in the National Assistance Board, the UN Secretariat in New York and the Cabinet Office, and later went to 10 Downing Street as Principal Private Secretary where, between 1975 and 1979, he served Harold Wilson, Jim Callaghan and Margaret Thatcher.

   He moved to the Northern Ireland office as Permanent Secretary in 1979. In 1981 he became Permanent Secretary at the DHSS. He retired a few weeks before Norman Fowler left the Department, but he maintained an active involvement in international and health affairs as, among other things, a non-executive director of the Royal Marsden Hospital. He was knighted in 1986.

Throughout the dispute the DHSS and the TUC kept their lines wide open. The leaders of the TUC were very lukewarm about the industrial action and wanted a clean settlement. Peter Jacques, who chaired the TUC Health Committee, and Albert Spanswick, the General Secretary of the Confederation of Health Service Employees, met Norman Fowler and Kenneth Stowe, the Permanent Secretary, at Fowler's house in Fulham on a regular basis. Often these meetings, which were 'off the record', lasted little more than an hour while, over a glass of whisky, they compared notes and explored their respective positions and room for manoeuvre.[29]

It was at one of these meetings, according to Ken Stowe, that the need for stronger and more professional management, especially management of personnel, in the NHS emerged. As winter approached the dispute began to run out of steam. By mid-November only 12% of health districts in England and Wales were experiencing significant action. The rest were back to normal working. Despite this, the conflict dragged on until December when, after a gruelling weekend in the DHSS headquarters at the Elephant and Castle in London, a final settlement was reached. It was far short of the claim, and what is more it was applied differentially. Nurses, midwives and health visitors got a pay review body, like the doctors and dentists.

The final settlement included an agreement to appoint an inquiry into the management of the NHS workforce.

Although both the DHSS and the trade unions may have seen such an inquiry as a genuine attempt to learn from the dispute and to make things better for the future, there was also a strong undercurrent of dissatisfaction inside the DHSS, among both ministers and officials, with the performance of some health authorities and their managers. In Birmingham, for example, some of the health authorities had struck a series of deals with local union leaders that protected emergency and urgent work. In return for this, the health authorities agreed not to admit non-urgent cases, to block private practice, not to open closed wards and not to use contractors to undertake duties normally undertaken by NHS staff. The DHSS view was that:

> These health authorities seem to be acquiescing in the breach of contract by their staff. Their surrender to the trade unions prevents them from employing other management responses such as calling in volunteers and contractors. If they make a move they become initiators of action and the unions the respondents – so they have lost important strategic, tactical and PR advantages.[30]

This was in Norman Fowler's own constituency territory, and as a result central intervention was problematic. There was a worry that 'any intervention from above could lead to strong and possibly damaging union reprisals. . . . Cannot hope to stiffen management's backbone in North Birmingham without implicating the Secretary of State to some degree or other.'[30]

In the summer of 1982, the MP Ralph Howell had also been asking the Prime Minister, Margaret Thatcher, for an inquiry into the NHS which had in his view 'no chairman or titular head and no one person in overall control of any Health Authority or Hospital'. Mrs Thatcher told Fowler at a meeting in October 1982 that she had great sympathy with his views and thought an inquiry might be a good idea.[31] She, like Howell, had been influenced by a series of articles in *The*

Daily Telegraph by Graham Turner in the autumn of 1982 which, Mrs Thatcher told Fowler, had revealed 'a total absence of effective management systems in the NHS.'[32]

Turner had argued that the most pressing need 'is to appoint a man of first-class ability to manage the NHS.'[33]

At this stage the NHS was still operating consensus-based management teams, with very variable success. From 1982 these teams were subject to close monitoring by the DHSS by means of a new and powerful performance-monitoring system, called the accountability process, which was initiated as a response to a critical report by the Public Accounts Committee in 1981. Once a year the chairman of each regional health authority was summoned to London with his team of officers to be grilled by the Secretary of State about their performance and future plans. 'What have you done with all the money invested in your region?' was a new and very challenging question, and it drew both ministers and officials very close to the heart of the management of the NHS. Each side prepared in great detail, and the conclusions of the meeting were published in an exchange of letters that were made public and included performance targets for the following year. Eventually this process was cascaded down the system, with regions holding DHAs to account in the same manner, and they in turn did the same with their operational units.

This system worked well in many parts of the NHS, but eventually ministers got bored with the process. The Secretary of State passed the task to his junior ministers, and the Permanent Secretary attended less and less frequently. The briefing papers continued to grow, and the final exchange of letters began to be drafted in advance and was sometimes negotiated in some detail weeks before the event. The process eventually developed into a complex performance management function in its own right with its myriad targets. The reality of accountability necessarily involved grappling with a lot of detail.

Finding Griffiths

The decision to launch a management inquiry was announced at the Conservative Party Conference in September 1982 and attracted little attention at the time. At this stage it was clear, at least to Fowler, that the focus of the inquiry would be on the non-medical staffing of the NHS and its management, although there was some disagreement about the purpose of the review even at this stage. Stowe remembers that 'Ken Clarke was wanting to have a manpower inquiry, whilst Roy, Norman and I were quite clear it was to be a management inquiry.'[2] What Fowler and Stowe wanted to secure was more efficient management of NHS manpower.

Fowler might have been tempted to have an ever more wide-ranging review, to include the wider policy territory of the whole basis of funding for the NHS. However, he judged that 'the pitch had been queered in 1973' when the Centre for Policy Studies (a Tory think tank) produced a report on this subject in what Fowler regarded as 'a classically bad way.'[29] The study had been undertaken without the knowledge of most ministers and then leaked to *The Economist*. It concluded that there was a case for the privatisation of the NHS. However, in Fowler's view 'no one was quite sure what that meant, including the authors.'[29]

The report caused a political storm and was quickly buried. Fowler did not want Griffiths straying into this dangerous territory, and therefore funding the NHS was not to be part of his brief. He was asked to work 'on the supposition and premise that the NHS remained a publicly financed service and financed in the same way.'[29]

Fowler's clear brief when he came into office was 'to make the NHS more efficient,'[29] and this included a move on competitive tendering for some ancillary services. Norman Fowler's view accorded closely with that of Margaret Thatcher, who could see that all was not well with the NHS but who was not yet ready for major reform or fundamental change.

Thatcher's view was as follows:

> The NHS was a huge organisation which inspired at least as much affection as exasperation, whose emergency services reassured even those who hoped they would not have to use them, and whose basic structure was felt by most people to be sound. Any reforms must not undermine public confidence.[34]

Inside the Department, officials were exploring options for the future, including some that would create distance between itself and the NHS. What blocked them at every stage was the issue of the accountability of the Secretary of State to Parliament. The phrase 'every time a maid kicks over a bucket of slops in a ward an agonised wail will go through Whitehall'[35] was by now a powerful principle that governed policies relating to the management of public services at a national level.

One of these exploratory papers prepared in September 1983 concluded that there was no satisfactory alternative to maintaining the position in which the Secretary of State was head and leader of the NHS. Attached to it is a handwritten note by Stowe, in an exchange with G G Hulme, the Principal Finance Officer for the Department, which states that 'there is one [i.e. an alternative] but it is too costly and requires legislation.'[32]

As usual, it was Kenneth Stowe who started to put the wheels in motion concerning the management inquiry. By December the Prime Minister was pressing for progress and hoped that 'somebody could be found who would not be too closely associated with the medical establishment.'[32] In fact, the front runner at this stage, Basil E C Collins, the Group Chief Executive of Cadbury Schweppes, was also the Chairman of the Finance and General Purposes Committee of the Royal College of Nursing, so he knew quite a lot about the NHS. However, after some thought he declined the offer on the grounds that the timing was wrong. An election was coming, the most recent NHS reorganisation was not completed, industrial relations had not settled down and the nursing profession in particular was focusing on the pay review body to the exclusion of everything else. He reported 'some cynicism about the purpose of an inquiry and expressed doubts about whether the Government meant business or not.'[32]

Stowe moved to the second choice. The name of Roy Griffiths had been put forward by Jonathan Charkham, an old contact in the City who at that time was the Director of PRO-NED, an organisation that promoted and supported non-executive directors.[2] He had been the Director of Public Appointments in the Civil Service Department until 1982. Roy Griffiths was the Deputy Chairman and Managing Director of Sainsbury's, the supermarket chain, and was rated by

Charkham as the best personnel management man in the country. John Sainsbury confirmed this opinion when approached by Stowe. Having cleared an approach with Norman Fowler, Stowe rang Griffiths and arranged a meeting at Sainsbury's headquarters in Stamford Street, London. To begin with Griffiths was cool, aloof and hostile. He gave Stowe a hard time but eventually agreed to chair a review. Stowe reported back to Fowler that Griffiths' 'main concern was that it should not be seen as a cost-cutting exercise, nor should it be assumed that greater efficiency would alone solve the service's problems. He would wish to be concerned with resources, placing primary emphasis on manpower.'[2] He may well have been influenced to chair the review by his family connections with the world of medicine.

Sir Ernest Roy Griffiths

Roy Griffiths was born on 8 July 1926 and was educated at Wolstanton Grammar School, Staffordshire, and Keble College, Oxford. He became Deputy Chairman of J Sainsbury Ltd in 1975 and Managing Director in 1979. Margaret Thatcher brought him in as part-time adviser to the NHS. He chaired the team that produced the *NHS Management Inquiry Report* (known as the Griffiths Report),[24] which was published in 1983, and contained the memorable phrase: 'If Florence Nightingale was carrying her lamp through the corridors of the NHS today she would almost certainly be searching for the people in charge'. His report on community care was published in 1986.[36,54] Griffiths became a member of the NHS Supervisory and Policy Boards, the Prime Minister's special adviser on healthcare management and vice-chairman of the NHS Management Board during the time when it was chaired by Tony Newton as Minister of Health. For a number of years Griffiths maintained an office and separate staff in Richmond House, the headquarters of the DHSS.

In response to personal enquiries by Stowe, Len Murray of the TUC suggested Michael Bett of British Telecom as a member, and Hector Laing, the Chairman of United Biscuits, suggested Jim Blyth, his Finance Director.[2] Sir Brian Bailey, Chairman of both Television South West and the Health Education Council, completed the team. The team was supported by an atypical civil servant called Cliff Graham who got on famously with Griffiths and had a good rapport with managers in the NHS.

The Sun newspaper announced the appointment to the NHS as 'Supermarket boss to head team of whizz-kids who will check out the NHS.'[37]

Terms of reference

Before they had even begun their inquiry, the early lack of consensus about the purpose of the inquiry caused difficulties when it came to agreeing the terms of reference. According to Kenneth Clarke, who was still the Minister for Health under Fowler, the inquiry was about manpower and how to manage and reduce it.[2] At the end of January he told Fowler 'I do feel we have got into a most unfortunate difficulty with Mr Griffiths. We are almost at cross-purposes with him.'[32]

Clarke was also 'a bit annoyed at first; my nose had been put slightly out of joint. I wasn't being allowed to form my own policy; some businessman was going to be forming it for me.'[38]

Griffiths continued to argue that the inquiry must be about management, and won the day. He had the support of Mrs Thatcher, who intervened in February 1983 with a note to Fowler:

> The Prime Minister believes that over-manning is only the symptom of bad management. Mr Fowler should make it clear to the inquiry that the central task is to take a searching look at those general manage-ment issues underlying our concerns. The chain of command within hospitals is the most important of these questions.[32]

Fowler was of the same mind:

> We were conscious that management was not the health service's strong suit at that stage, and we were also conscious of the fact that we didn't have management skills actually inside the Department of Health itself. If you compared Health with Social Security, which I was in a very good position to do, Social Security had experience of direct management, they did manage the whole outfit, they managed the Benefit Shops and the rest and they were responsible for it. That was not the case on the health side; they didn't really manage anything, they were advisers to me and to the Health Service.[29]

A review that had started out with the intention of concentrating on workforce and personnel issues had, according to Graham Hart, later to become Permanent Secretary, been 'transmuted into something which was rather different, which was how to manage the NHS in a much broader sense.'[39]

The Griffiths Report

During the course of the inquiry, Griffiths and his team received advice from many quarters, with the majority inside the NHS arguing for something close to the status quo. A few, including Ralph Howells MP, urged Griffiths to consider recommending an independent corporation. Of particular interest is a back-ground paper prepared by N J B Evans on behalf of the leading civil servants inside the DHSS, which reached the following conclusion:

> In summary, although the Department exercises many of the func-tions of a head office of the NHS, it does not act as a manager of the NHS in the full sense of the word. Ministers control financial resources for the NHS and appointments to regional health authorities and the chairmen of DHAs. They have statutory powers of direction, albeit rarely used. DHSS officers, acting on behalf of ministers, can exercise significant influence over the management of NHS affairs. They have no line relationship with NHS officers, nor do most of them possess any detailed expertise in the running of health services. The Department has seen it as its job to provide a broad steer on policies and priorities to

the NHS and the resources to follow it, to ensure the regions keep within these resources and do not stray far off course in policy terms. It has not seen its job, nor is it equipped to intervene in the detailed operations of the NHS, or to manage the one million staff employed.[40]

When it was published in October 1983, the Griffiths Report was much praised for its simplicity, conciseness (25 pages) and directness.[24] It was also launched with a memorable phrase, attributed to Cliff Graham, which caught the headlines: 'In short, if Florence Nightingale were carrying her lamp through the corridors of the NHS today she would almost certainly be searching for the people in charge.' The report recommended the introduction of general management into the NHS. On Stowe's advice, recommendations that might require primary legislation were avoided so that they could proceed quickly within the existing statutory framework.

The inquiry's terms of reference had not included a review of the organisation of the Department of Health, but the report nevertheless proposed major change at the headquarters.

As secretary to the inquiry, Cliff Graham had a substantial influence over the shape of the Griffiths Report. As one of his colleagues put it, 'there was a strong coincidence between what I knew to be Cliff's views and what appears in the Griffiths Report.'[39]

A new style of management: the Griffiths Report 1983[24]

- The creation of a Health Service Supervisory Board (HSSB) within the Department of Health and Social Security and the existing statutory framework, which would be chaired by the Secretary of State. The Board's role would be to determine the purpose, objectives and direction of the health service, to approve the overall budget and resource allocations, to take strategic decisions and to receive reports on performance and other evaluations within the health service.

- The setting up of a small, multi-professional NHS Management Board (NHSMB), accountable to the Supervisory Board, to plan the implementation of policies, give leadership to the management of the NHS, control performance and achieve consistency and drive over the long term. The Board would have members drawn from business, the NHS and the Civil Service. Its chairman would perform the general management role at a national level and also act as accounting officer for health service expenditure.

- General managers to be appointed at all levels of the NHS with the freedom to organise their management structures in the way best suited to local requirements.

- The appointment of a Director of Personnel at Management Board level, drawn from outside the NHS to lead the development of personnel relations.

- A powerful push for devolution and a greater involvement by clinicians, who would manage their own budgets.

Implementing the Griffiths Report

Fowler considered the Griffiths Report to be excellent,[29] and accepted its main thrust and recommendations and sent it out for consultation. The Prime Minister and the Cabinet also liked the conclusions of the report.[29] It had a mixed reception within the NHS, as Griffiths himself reflected nearly ten years later:

> The nurses saw it as a challenge to a carefully established professional career structure. The medical profession saw the report correctly as questioning whether their clinical autonomy extended to immunity from being questioned as to how resources were being used. All the professions saw the report as introducing economics into the care of patients, believing this was inimical to good care.[41]

At the time, even within the DHSS, there were those with doubts and with concerns that the emphasis on management would weaken the policy-making role. Graham Hart, who was later to become Permanent Secretary, was at this stage leading the team considering how to reorganise the DHSS in the light of the Griffiths Report. He reported to Stowe that 'the word management can lead to some confusion when one is considering the Department's activities in respect of the NHS. Some say that the Department does not in any real sense manage the NHS and could not do so without reform of the statutory framework.'[26]

Others inside the Department saw the new Board as little more than a focus for discussion of issues relating to NHS management. Members of the Board would remain accountable for their departments, and professional members would continue to look to their head of profession.[42] One way of achieving this was to ensure that the chairman and each member of the team had a portfolio of their own for which they were personally responsible. This would avoid the possibility of the chairman acting like a Prime Minister served by his own immediate staff.[32] Others distinguished the chairman from his board by assuming that 'it was the job of the Chairman of the Management Board to translate into management action the decisions reached in the HSSB.'[43]

The trade unions were most unhappy at what they perceived as their lack of involvement in the Griffiths Inquiry, which is somewhat ironic given its roots. They doubted the need to look outside the NHS or the Civil Service for any of the key appointments. The Royal College of Nursing was scathing in its criticism, and its representative body deeply deplored the implications for healthcare and the nursing profession. The doctors were predictably negative, with the medical Royal Colleges saying that the general reaction was one of fear, in particular that the establishment of a general manager would restrict change and damage the progress made over recent years in the status and responsibility of the professions' senior managers. The Faculty of Community Medicine reflected a common concern about yet another reorganisation occurring so soon after the last one.

The Chief Medical Officer (CMO), Donald Acheson, was in private at least more constructive, and advised Stowe that even if it did assume 'that hospitals were the only thing that mattered', the report, if implemented, could 'transform the NHS for the better'. His was the only significant voice to wonder about the respective roles of the Supervisory and Management Boards. His instincts told him that 'one would matter and the other would not.'[40] Acheson, like Stowe, was always conscious of the Department's wider contribution to government policy formulation. 'The structure of these Boards should also take into account the need for better liaison with Social Security and the Department of the Environment in respect of housing.' He argued that 'This was particularly relevant to the care of the elderly, which will be one of the greatest problems to be faced by health services in the next 20 years, and in which the nature of the accommodation provided is the key to both care and cost.'[40] He also pressed for doctors to be made eligible to be appointed to the new general manager posts.[40]

Regional chairmen welcomed the report and were confident that their role would not be diminished. The CMO provided confirmation of this in a note to Stowe following a discussion with the regional chairmen in October 1983. This meeting convinced him that the new Chairman and his Management Board could not have a powerful new management function. The Director General (as the job was called at this stage in the discussions) would not have a line-management relationship with regional health authorities or their officers. 'What is left,' the CMO pondered, 'except for an advisory role?'[44] 'This is not,' he pointed out, 'how others, including the Prime Minister, see the role'.

The Opposition, led by Michael Meacher, was very sceptical. Meacher wrote to Norman Fowler on 9 January 1984: 'Given six weeks, including Christmas and New Year, this is not an exercise in consultation, it is a cynical piece of manipulation. You are just trying to make NHS management the scapegoats for the NHS failing.'[45] Gwyneth Dunwoody was just as critical: 'General managers who will override the clinical judgements of the medical establishment and tell nurses that their background reviews on the staffing of hospital wards and theatres do not matter.'[46]

Despite the reservations of many, including the Health Select Committee of the House of Commons, the Government proceeded with implementation.

A new Supervisory Board was established in October 1983.

Membership of the Health Service Supervisory Board

Chairman: Secretary of State	Norman Fowler
Minister of State	Tony Newton and
	later Kenneth Clarke
Parliamentary Secretary (Health)	John Patton
Parliamentary Secretary (Lords)	Lord Glenarthur
Permanent Secretary	Kenneth Stowe
Chief Medical Officer	Henry Yellowlees
Chief Nursing Officer	Anne Poole
Independent member	Roy Griffiths

The HSSB met for the first time on 22 December 1983, almost a year before Paige was appointed, and met pretty much on a monthly basis until March 1987. Kenneth Stowe organised the early meetings and personally briefed Norman Fowler, the Secretary of State, prior to each meeting.

The role of the Board was clearly delineated in the minutes of the first meeting as being 'To support ministers in considering major strategy issues. The establishment of the Board did not alter the statutory responsibilities of ministers or their formal relationships with health authorities. The Board itself had no corporate status: the decisions were all for the Secretary of State.'[47] This was a somewhat paler version of the model recommended by Griffiths, who had seen its role as the determination of strategy, the allocation of resources and the evaluation of NHS performance.

It was in reality to be a high-level sounding board that provided a focus for policy making by ministers. It was not supposed to play any part in the day-to-day management of the NHS. With the Secretary of State in the chair it no doubt had a substantial influence on the affairs of the NHS as well as the wider Department of Health.

Stowe's guidelines for the management of the Supervisory Board[47]

- The papers to be confidential and numbered.
- Issued only to members, and no photocopies to be made.
- Minutes to be terse and impersonal (Cabinet Office style).
- Each item to conclude with Secretary of State's decision.
- Minutes would not record that Board 'took note' or 'agreed'.
- Dates of meetings not to be publicised.

Meetings were normally held at the headquarters of the DHSS at the Elephant and Castle, and usually started in the late afternoon. On a few occasions the Board met at the House of Commons.

Victor Paige joined the Supervisory Board in January 1985 as Chairman of the NHS Management Board. The Board met regularly during the first two years of its existence. The business of the first year was inevitably dominated by the implementation of the Griffiths Report, but as that year progressed and into the next, other issues gained a slot on the agenda. The Supervisory Board ended in June 1988 and met only six times in the last two years of its life.

The table opposite shows a summary of business conducted by the Supervisory Board in the 17 meetings from December 1983 to December 1985.[48]

Preparing for change at the centre

While the search for the first chairman of the NHS Management Board continued in earnest, an Interim Management Board pushed on with the detailed preparations. Stowe, however, warned his colleagues 'not to rush to make changes to Departmental structures in case the new Chief Executive does not like it, and the NHS may be very suspicious of changes at this stage.'[45]

Patrick Benner, deputy secretary and another member of Stowe's senior team, put the issue squarely to his colleagues in November, saying:

> The reality is that, at the top level, decisions will be taken by the Secretary of State with the advice of the HSSB; and that at a lower level, decisions will be made by the Chairman of the Management Board, perhaps after discussion with all members of the Board or perhaps after talking to only one or two. My point is whether we are

	Topic	Meeting(s) in which it was discussed
1	Role and structure of the Supervisory Board and the Management Board	1, 4, 5, 11, 12, 14, 16, 17
2	Implementation of the Griffiths Report	1, 2, 3, 4, 5, 6
3	Pay and industrial relations	2, 8
4	Development of primary care	1, 2, 7, 9
5	Review of NHS strategic plans	2, 3
6	Competitive tendering for support services in hospitals	5, 8, 9, 13
7	Medical manpower	7, 10
8	Public expenditure survey	3, 17
9	Rayner efficiency studies	4, 5, 6, 10, 13
10	NHS manpower targets/personnel strategy	5, 6, 8
11	DHSS restructuring	7
12	Warnock Report	7
13	Food Hygiene at Stanley Royd Hospital Report	8
14	Care of the elderly	1, 2, 10, 14
15	Private patient charges	9
16	Nursing priorities	10, 11
17	Report on the NHS	6
18	Medical Research Council grants	7
19	General managers	8
20	Performance indicators	11
21	Health promotion and disease	11, 12
22	Unit general management	12
23	Community care	13
24	Limited list medicines	13, 16
25	NHS purchasing	14
26	Residential accommodation	15
27	Personal social services	15
28	Acquired immune deficiency syndrome (AIDS)	16
29	Community medicine	17
30	McColl Report: Artificial Limb and Appliance Centres (ALAC)	17

going to present and talk about the new arrangement as though the constitutional position is different from what it actually is.[40]

Stowe took soundings within Whitehall about the definition of the Chairman's role, all of which seemed to confirm the sanctity of the Secretary of State's position. The consensus among senior civil servants across Whitehall was that the Secretary of State cannot delegate his responsibility to Parliament to anyone.[40]

The Treasury was also heavily involved and was looking for 'the new functions, roles and accountabilities of individuals to be defined as closely as possible'. The Treasury sought 'maximum clarity.'[40]

Fowler and Clarke also found themselves having to get to grips with the detail of this new animal that they were creating. The question was raised as to whether it was intended to create a Board which appeared as near as possible to a separate corporation within the existing statutory framework. 'No,' Fowler replied, 'any attempt to present the Board as a corporation in embryo would be a fiction and quickly identified as such.'[43]

In October 1983 Stowe told his colleagues that the 'Secretary of State had agreed that regional chairmen will remain directly accountable to him and not to any Chief Executive or Director General.'[40] On 29 November 1983 the detail was finally settled, and Fowler told Stowe to get ahead quickly 'on the clear understanding that there is no question of creating an independent body with corporate status, and that appointees would work on behalf of and under the authority of the Secretary of State as other civil servants do.'[43]

Even before Paige was appointed, difficulties were emerging with the Treasury about the pay and grading of the new management team, which had to sit within existing Civil Service pay structures. A leading Regional Administrator, Michael Fairey, was drafted in to help with a study of the traffic flows between the Department of Health and the NHS. Griffiths was strongly in favour of bringing NHS managers into the DHSS, as was David Owen, a former Minister of Health, who urged Fowler to 'bridge the gap between the civil service in the Elephant and Castle, and the health administrators in the regions and districts who understood the management of the NHS and should bring them on to the Management Board and into the DHSS.'[45] Stowe was more cautious, and had a worried staff to placate. He expressed to his colleagues 'a concern that the NHS has not got to get the impression that there are a lot of well-paid jobs at the centre earmarked for them.'[49]

One exchange with Don Wilson, the Chairman of the Mersey RHA, captured the mood when he was asked to agree to the secondment of his Treasurer to the DHSS. He responded as follows:

> You will be aware of the prominence of both Everton and Liverpool in the Milk Cup [football]. We have not talked about transfer fees or loan recognition. I am sure that in view of the high figures for people of high professional ability in this area, you will be mindful of this in your discussions. I know he can score goals.[50]

The reply was as follows:

> My association these days is with Ipswich Town, who got into some difficulty in this matter, but your point is well made and we have it very much in mind.[50]

When the official circular about the implementation of the Griffiths Inquiry in the NHS was issued, it turned out to be very much more prescriptive than had been expected. Stowe had worried about this himself as he worked on it. Finding the right balance between laissez-faire and over-prescription 'had been difficult,' he told Fowler. He was particularly worried about 'another premature retirement fiasco'[2] which had attracted so much adverse criticism on the last occasion when the NHS had been reorganised.

The first step in the reorganisation plan was to sort out the regional health authorities and reconstitute their boards so that they could proceed to appoint their own general managers. Up and down the country the most senior managers in the NHS began to apply for general manager posts (not at this stage labelled chief executive). The first stage of competition was limited to members of the existing regional teams, and only if a satisfactory candidate could not be found was the search extended. By the late summer of 1984 most regional appointments had been made. For the most part they went to the incumbent administrator, but two went to medicine and one to nursing.[51] They were all on short-term contracts (usually three years) and performance-related pay. In each case the regional chairman had to clear his proposed appointment with the Secretary of State before it could be confirmed.

At a district level the same process cascaded down. In the DHSS there was real concern that the administrators would pick up all the jobs and nothing would really change. Ministers and the Supervisory Board kept an anxious count as the results rolled in. In the event, about 60% of the jobs went to administrators and the balance was split among doctors, nurses, business and men and women of the armed forces.

All of this was well in hand before Paige, who was to be the first NHS Chief Executive, was appointed. He had little opportunity to influence the selection of the first wave of general managers in the NHS.

Dialogue with the deaf

In the search for clarity about the NHS at this point in its history, it is important to remember the financial restraints under which it was forced to operate. Public expenditure had been squeezed hard, real growth rates were very low and pay restraint was the dominant feature of relationships with the trade unions. As Fowler explains, 'public spending was under severe restraint and you had to fight for every bit of extra resource you got, and you had to prove that any you did secure was used effectively'. At this stage, he explains, 'we were responsible for 40% of all public expenditure, and if a Chancellor wished to reduce public spending, guess where he came to.'[29]

Fowler claims that the professions never understood this:

> They were opposed to virtually every change. It was not a matter of 'making it more efficient, Secretary of State', just a question of 'more resources, more resources'. All they wanted was a higher level of investment. It was a dialogue with the deaf.[29]

Chapter 2

Timeline

1985

- Victor Paige was appointed as first Chairman of the NHS Management Board on 2 January. Mrs Thatcher urged him to 'approach the task with vigour.'
- Ian Mills was appointed from Price Waterhouse as Finance Director.
- The Project 2000 group was appointed by the UK Central Council for Nursing, Midwifery and Health Visiting to review the training of nurses, midwives and health visitors.
- The miners called off their national strike.
- Family health service authorities were established as statutory bodies in April.
- *Reflections on the Management of the NHS* (the Enthoven Report)[52] was published, which recommended the introduction of an internal market into the NHS.
- Stowe wrote to Fowler with outline proposals for an English health authority.
- Regional General Manager Duncan Nichol joined the national NHS Management Board.
- In November, Len Peach was appointed Personnel Director of the NHS Management Board.
- Fowler objected to the Management Board 'deciding' anything. He made it plain that their role was to offer advice to ministers.

January to June 1986

- A report[53] was published of the inquiry into the outbreak of salmonella poisoning at the Stanley Royd Hospital. This criticised management at all levels, from the hospital to the RHA.
- In April, the Greater London Council and Metropolitan Counties were abolished.
- The Chernobyl nuclear accident occurred.
- Ian Mills launched the Management Accountancy Framework and sought to draw doctors into the management of their budgets.
- On 3 June, Victor Paige resigned as Chairman of the NHS Management Board.
- Len Peach took over as acting Chairman of the Management Board until November, when it was restructured with the Minister of Health (Tony Newton) in the chair.
- The Green Paper *Community Care: an Agenda for Discussion*[54] was published.

Victor Paige, 1985–86

It was Kenneth Stowe who led the hunt for the first chairman of the NHS Management Board. Five firms of headhunters were interviewed in March 1984, and these were quickly reduced to two. PA Personnel Services was eventually appointed, and the first advertisement appeared in the press in April 1984.[55]

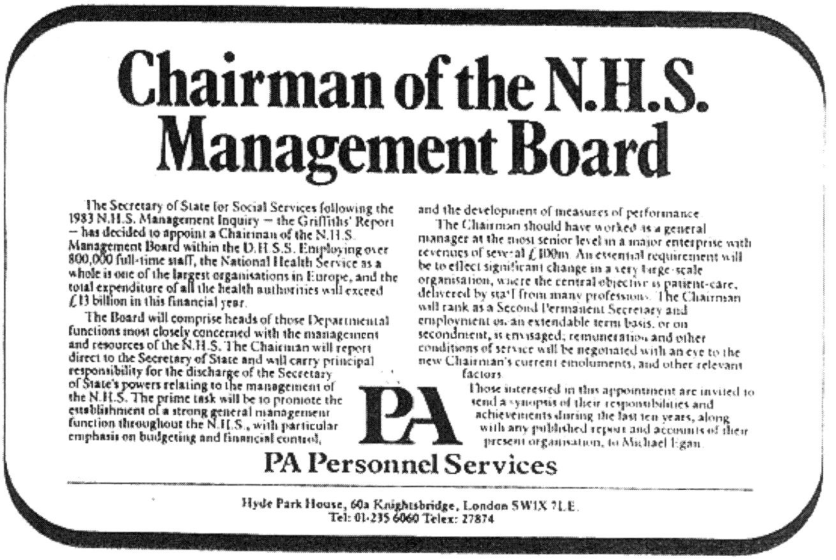

Chairman of the N.H.S. Management Board

The Secretary of State for Social Services following the 1983 N.H.S. Management Inquiry – the Griffiths' Report – has decided to appoint a Chairman of the N.H.S. Management Board within the D.H.S.S. Employing over 800,000 full-time staff, the National Health Service as a whole is one of the largest organisations in Europe, and the total expenditure of all the health authorities will exceed £13 billion in this financial year.

The Board will comprise heads of those Departmental functions most closely concerned with the management and resources of the N.H.S. The Chairman will report direct to the Secretary of State and will carry principal responsibility for the discharge of the Secretary of State's powers relating to the management of the N.H.S. The prime task will be to promote the establishment of a strong general management function throughout the N.H.S., with particular emphasis on budgeting and financial control,

and the development of measures of performance.

The Chairman should have worked as a general manager at the most senior level in a major enterprise with revenues of several £100m. An essential requirement will be to effect significant change in a very large-scale organisation, where the central objective is patient-care, delivered by staff from many professions. The Chairman will rank as a Second Permanent Secretary and employment on an extendable term basis, or on secondment, is envisaged; remuneration and other conditions of service will be negotiated with an eye to the new Chairman's current emoluments, and other relevant factors.

Those interested in this appointment are invited to send a synopsis of their responsibilities and achievements during the last ten years, along with any published report and accounts of their present organisation, to Michael Egan.

PA

PA Personnel Services

Hyde Park House, 60a Knightsbridge, London SW1X 7LE.
Tel: 01-235 6060 Telex: 27874

Figure 2.1

The advertisement and job description did not please everybody in Whitehall. The Downing Street Efficiency Unit considered that it was 'very much a description of a Civil Service job', and they questioned whether it would attract top people. They thought that the advertisement was not pitched in terms of 'wanting someone special to achieve something special.'[56]

They wanted the chairman to be seen as the Secretary of State's right-hand man who would be 'seen to speak for him'. They were worried that the present advertisement signalled 'As you were.'[56] Downing Street clearly had in mind a big player who could turn the troubled NHS around. Stowe had a rather different image in mind. In an exchange with the Treasury in January 1984 he explained:

> it is vital that the candidates reading this job description should in no circumstances be led to believe that they are being recruited as general manager of the NHS. There is not, and cannot be under the existing law, a person holding that office within the DHSS, and I think we put the whole Griffiths exercise in relation to the NHS at risk if we attempt to promote a bogus prospectus.[56]

Stowe later told Sir Robert Armstrong that the new chairman needed:

> to combine the ability to work effectively and at a very senior level within a government department with experience and skill in effecting change in a necessarily decentralised organisation.[43]

Paige recalls one official telling him that the first draft made it explicit that the appointment did not involve the chairman and directors taking and implementing decisions, and that their powers were limited to offering advice to ministers. He did not believe the story at the time.[57]

Despite a flurry of early interest, the results were disappointing. Over 60 candidates were sifted down to three by the middle of June, and these were interviewed on 9 September 1984 on neutral ground at the Royal Institute of Chartered Surveyors in London. There was much discussion about the venue for these interviews. The Athenaeum Club was eventually felt to be too public, and the Old Admiralty Building and Stowe's office were considered to be inappropriate.

Roy Griffiths was not to be involved in the final interview process, so that the position would be safeguarded in the event that he decided to apply.

Analysis of the applicants for the post of Chairman of the NHS Management Board[58]

Sector

Engineering	10
Public sector	11
Food and drink industry	5
Doctors and dentists	5
Oil industry	4
Chemical industry	4
Business consultants	3
Other industries	14

The long list included a substantial majority with boardroom experience. The average age was just over 50 years. There was one woman.

All of the short-listed candidates had impressive industrial credentials, but none was judged by the panel to be above the line and suitable for appointment. One, from a major engineering company, was judged not to have the force of personality or resourcefulness required. The second candidate, from the Institute of Directors, seemed to lack the leadership qualities required. The third candidate, from a major oil company, had openly agonised about whether the job could be done, and in any case wanted more money than was ever likely to be available.[57]

Final interview panel[59]

Mr Dennis Trevelyan, First Civil Service Commissioner
Sir Kenneth Stowe, Permanent Secretary
Dr Donald Acheson, Chief Medical Officer
Professor Robert Whelan, Vice-Chancellor, University of Liverpool, and doctor
Sir Robin Ibbs, Downing Street Efficiency Unit

The process stalled and the headhunters quietly withdrew. Kenneth Stowe and Sir Robert Armstrong, Head of the Home Civil Service, tried another trawl among the leaders of industry, and this time they were prepared to consider a secondment. These approaches produced some interest, including a number of elderly but distinguished medical peers, but no result. A frank internal appraisal of the process in January 1985 is interesting for its conclusion that the 'people of the calibre required were likely to be either too expensive and possibly too high-profile, or affordable but reluctant to leave the private sector for fear of falling behind their peers.' The result of all this was that the natural catchment group was composed 'of the unemployed, those who were not of the calibre required, or those nearing the end of their careers but who had not been successful enough to be out of reach financially.'[60]

By November 1984 *The Sunday Times* reported that there were no takers for the £60 000 job as head of the NHS.[61] MPs began to raise their concerns. John Redwood MP, who was later to run for the leadership of the Conservative Party, wrote to Norman Fowler in December pressing for:

> [the] Chairman to have powers in relation to medical staff, powers to appoint staff in the NHS, powers to set service standards and budgets as well as powers to take action against ineffective management in the NHS.[56]

As the delay in making an appointment extended, other voices began to intrude. Both *The Daily Mail* and *The Sunday Times* reported that the new post had infuriated civil servants who believed that they should have had a chance to compete for the job. The feeling was that you could not run the health service like a factory or a firm of stockbrokers. They thought that a job like this needed a great deal of experience, which only a top civil servant could acquire.

Meanwhile Norman Fowler and Kenneth Clarke had been making their own enquiries. Both knew Victor Paige from their days at the Ministry of Transport. Paige had been the Personnel Director and Deputy Chairman of the National Freight Corporation, and had been persuaded by them to become Chairman of the Port of London Authority. Fowler rang Paige at home late one Tuesday evening and suggested meeting for breakfast at Browns Hotel two days later.[62] On Thursday of the same week Fowler, who was accompanied by Kenneth Clarke, opened the conversation by explaining that he was hunting for a chairman of the new NHS Management Board. Paige had read about the Griffiths Report in the newspapers, but at this stage his knowledge was slight. The three men talked for nearly three hours and they were the last to leave the dining room. According to Paige it had been an interesting conversation, but he had left with many questions in his mind. He understood what a powerful job it was: 'the biggest managerial job in the country, probably in the world, and you cannot just tell a Secretary of State to take a running jump.'[62] In any case he had respect for Fowler and Clarke based on his earlier dealings with them. He said that he would think about it, and went back to his office. To his astonishment he found a letter waiting for him from Fowler asking him to consider the matter very seriously and hoping that he would accept the job. Enclosed with the letter was a copy of the Griffiths Report.

Victor Paige, Chief Executive of the NHS, 1985–86[62]

Victor Paige was born in East Ham in 1925, the son of a docker. He attended the local grammar school and volunteered for RAF Air Crew service on his seventeenth birthday in 1942, but was not called up until 1943. He got early release in 1947 and went to Nottingham University to read social science.

While he was there he met the Personnel Director of Boots the Chemists, who later offered him a job within the Company's personnel department. While at Boots he held a Roosevelt Memorial Scholarship and spent several months in the USA.

He left Boots in 1967 and took over the personnel function at the Co-operative Wholesale Society in Manchester, which was undergoing massive management changes. He stayed for 'three fascinating years'.

His next post was as Director of Personnel at the newly created National Freight Corporation (NFC) in London, where he rapidly rose to Deputy Chairman and was deeply involved in the privatisation of the Company in 1981. At the NFC he was in close contact with Norman Fowler as Minister of Transport, and with Kenneth Clarke his deputy.

During 1980, Fowler asked him to consider becoming chairman of the Port of London Authority (PLA). Paige had doubts, mainly because of his father's background, but decided that he could do what had to be done more humanely than anyone else. He decided to accept, but insisted that it was a fifty-fifty job with the NFC. The job involved the closure of the Upper Thames Docks (including the docks where his father had worked), and this was achieved without any strikes.

In 1984 Fowler invited Paige to be chairman of the NHS Management Board. He took up the appointment on 2 January 1985 and resigned on 3 June 1986.

Paige decided to speak to Roy Griffiths and was encouraged by Fowler to speak to Kenneth Stowe.

At the first meeting at Browns Hotel with the ministers, Paige had asked questions about the management structure. He was not impressed by the explanations he received, and he thought that the proposals were 'ridiculous'. He was particularly concerned about the accountability of regional and district chairmen. He was surprised that district chairmen reported directly to ministers and not through the regional chairmen. From his perspective in industry he wondered 'What the hell are they playing at?'. He thought from the beginning that chairmen should be accountable directly to him rather than to ministers.[62] He was perplexed and puzzled about the role of the Supervisory Board, although Stowe and the interim team were already very clear that it was limited to an advisory role to the Secretary of State.

Ministers assured Paige that there would be no problem in sorting out the relationship between him and the regional chairmen. They would make sure that the chairmen were accountable to Paige, but they could not make this formal, as this would require primary legislation. Fowler assured Paige that 'you will take management decisions and I will make sure that you do.'[62] What he did not tell Paige was that he had agreed in October 1983 that regional chairmen would remain accountable to him and not to any chief executive or director general. It is most likely that Fowler had forgotten this promise, but the regional chairmen had not.

Paige's meeting with Stowe went well, but Stowe had been very direct with Paige about the accountability chain, the impossibility of primary legislation and the fact that at the end of the day all decisions would be made by ministers. It is more than likely that others who were working on Paige, including Cliff Graham, might have suggested that there was more room for manoeuvre on this issue than was in fact the case.

At this stage Paige also explored what it would mean in practice to be a Permanent Secretary (Grade 2) and accounting officer for the Health and Personal Social Services (HPSS) vote, which was huge. Stowe as First Permanent Secretary remained accounting officer for community and primary care, the four special hospitals and other headquarter services.

In retrospect, Paige regrets accepting the chairmanship on the basis of a Civil Service appointment. He explains:

> One of the reasons for the confusion relates to the decision to appoint the chairman as a second Permanent Secretary. I am not aware of the reasoning behind that, but believe it was cultivated by the Civil Service moguls who perhaps would have wished to retain the chairmanship of this unusual body within the civil service.[57]

Discussions inside the Department about the shape and structure of Paige's empire had been in progress for some time, and a management group led by Dr John Evans had been operating as an Interim Management Board since February 1984. It had been agreed with the Treasury that the Management Board would be accountable for the main NHS allocation (named Vote 1) but not for the Family Practitioner Services (FPS), on the grounds that some FPS issues were clearly political rather than managerial.[63] Stowe explained the decisions to exclude certain areas from the management arena as follows:

> The NHS is much more than health authorities. Don't forget that when the NHS Management Board was first set up, all the general practice side was outwith its remit – the enormous manpower surge was worrying everybody, including ministers, the administrators, the Treasury. The problem was seen as health authorities, the management of which was a problem. There wasn't the same concern about General Practice and Family Practitioner Committees.[2]

Interestingly, this change had prompted a debate about whether regional general managers should become accounting officers and thereby be accountable personally to the Public Accounts Committee. The matter was not pursued. There were worries among officials about a weakening of central control, the lack of experience among managers in being accountable to Parliament, and the possibility of creating own goals for the Secretary of State. In any case it was judged that the Public Accounts Committee would prefer 'a central bottom to kick.'[63] (This was of course to change later as chief executives of health organisations became accounting officers from 1995.) By this time Paige was getting 'twitchy'.[62] He now understood the onerous responsibilities of the accounting officer, but could not see that he had any managerial powers or controls to go with them. The best he had was the ability to commend to ministers. He would never have, as he put it, 'the power to take decisions in his hands.'[62, 64]

Paige continued the discussions with Fowler and Clarke into October 1984, when he went on holiday to Egypt. It was time for a decision. He was 59 years old and had planned his retirement from the Port of London Authority for the following year.

On the cruise boat down the Nile he sat at dinner with two American doctors. One was a medical school dean who had worked for two years in Windsor, so knew a fair amount about how the NHS operated. Paige explained his dilemma and passed over a copy of the Griffiths Report. The following day, instead of visiting temples they sat on deck and talked. It helped Paige to clear his mind. On his return he had more meetings about the degree of autonomy that he would have, his degree of management control and authority and the lines of accountability. He again met the block of primary legislation, but accepted with some reluctance Fowler and Clarke's assurance that there would be 'no problems: they would see to that.'[62]

Paige decided to accept on two conditions – first, that ministers honoured their promises with regard to his authority, and secondly, that he could retain a non-executive role as deputy chairman with the National Freight Corporation.

His appointment was announced in January 1985.

Paige chaired his first meeting of the Interim Team on 25 February 1985, when the continued confusion between the roles of the Board and the regions was aired. At this meeting they also shaped the agendas for future business. They wanted regular reports on the regions, monthly reports on the action taken to follow through on Rayner Efficiency Studies, regular reports on pay negotiations and waiting lists, and copies of the minutes of the national medical and nursing advisory committees. 'They did not need,' they considered, 'regular reports on NHS cash flow except on an exceptional basis.'[65]

Paige's first task was to assemble a management team, although a nucleus of civil servants was already in place on the Interim Board. Stowe had already put out feelers about secondments from industry. It took six months and some tough negotiations with the Treasury to appoint people from outside the system. Ian Mill's appointment as Director of Finance was particularly troublesome in terms of both salary and status. He was a senior partner with Price Waterhouse (one of four firms which had been approached for names),[50] and had a salary far in excess of any senior civil servant. 'Was he filling a permanent civil service post?' (and thereby counted against the Departmental open structure score), the Treasury asked 'or was he a consultant to the Board?'.[66] In the end a secondment deal was struck for a period of three years.

The appointment of a Director of Personnel was also problematic. The head-hunters Goddard, Kay and Rogers had advertised the post in April 1985, and final interviews took place in July and involved both Paige and Bett from the Griffiths team. There were four external candidates, from IBM, Philips, Imperial Tobacco and GEC, respectively. Len Peach from IBM, who had a very good reputation in the personnel management field but almost no industrial relations experience, was the successful candidate and took up post on 4 November 1985. He also came on secondment.

This issue of the salary and status of Board members from outside the Civil Service was to recur time and time again. It was not until some ten years later in 1996 that the issues were grasped and the posts were fully assimilated into Civil Service structures.

There was also a touch of interference from Number 10, who wanted to know why the NHS Management Board needed nine members when ICI managed very well with five. At stake was the second finance post on the Board. In the end Mrs Thatcher backed off, but Paige had not been best pleased with what he regarded as unnecessary political interference.[62]

The Chief Medical Officer accepted an invitation to join the Management Board, but only after some reflection. His brief, like Stowe's, was wider than the NHS, and he did not want to be accountable to Paige as were the other members of the Board. He joined the Supervisory Board as well. He did not want the Secretary of State to be receiving medical advice from more than one source.

Paige's first Management Board

Chairman	Victor Paige
Director of Operations and Vice-Chairman	Graham Hart (Civil Servant)
Public Sector Finance	Terri Banks (Civil Servant)
Corporate Finance	Ian Mills (Price Waterhouse)
Planning and IT	Mike Fairey (formerly Regional Administrator)
Regional Liaison	Cliff Graham (Civil Servant and Secretary to Griffiths Inquiry)
Doctor	Donald Acheson (Chief Medical Officer)
Nurse	Anne Poole (Chief Nursing Officer)
Personnel	Len Peach
Non-Executive Director	Duncan Nichol (Regional Manager, Mersey)
Property Adviser to the Board	Idris Pearce (part-time)
Director of Procurement and Distribution	Tom Critchley (from 2 January 1986)

The predominance of civil servants on the first Board drew much critical comment, but Paige himself thought the balance was about right.[67] The Board first met formally on 1 April 1985.

The principal interface role with the NHS at this time was through the Regional Liaison post, which was occupied by Cliff Graham, the civil servant who had been Secretary to the Griffiths Inquiry and who took upon himself the role of guardian of the Griffiths principles.

However, he did not survive long in that role and was succeeded by Anthony Merifield in November 1985. In the view of his Civil Service colleagues, Graham had become too committed and involved in the change process. 'He wanted to keep writing a new chapter.'[2] His passion for change was both his strength and his weakness.

At this stage Paige had 795 staff reporting directly to him, although he declared his intention to do with fewer.

In January 1985, Paige was able to present an upbeat progress report to the HSSB.[68]

The overall aims of the Management Board were summarised as being:

- to bring about continuing improvements in health services to patients. and to secure the implementation of the Secretary of State's service priorities
- to provide authoritative and challenging leadership to health authorities and their managers
- to ensure that health authorities have an adequate supply of well-trained and well-motivated staff
- to achieve a visible and positive impact on the perception of the NHS by the public, by its staff and by Parliament.

The planned action points were strong on financial control mechanisms, performance measures, efficiency and value for money, as well as better liaison with local government and the private sector. A review of resource allocations to NHS authorities was proposed, as was a big push to develop the quality of the finance function in the NHS. Manpower controls were to be maintained, with a continued push to reduce administrative and clerical staffing and shift the balance towards front-line staff. The NHS estate was targeted for rationalisation (with huge projected financial gains), as was the supplies function. Efficiency was seen to be at the heart of the Management Board's role.

Paige's early months were spent sorting out general managers' contracts and pay, preparing for the next general pay round, reacting to a raft of efficiency reports and assimilating the early products of performance management reports. The first tranche of general managers at regional and district level had been selected, but 700 unit managers still had to be appointed in the early part of 1986. Paige expected the number of doctors in management to be small at the start, but to grow over time.[69]

At their meeting in July 1985 the Management Board discussed the Enthoven Report,[52] which had proposed an internal market for the NHS. Paige thought that it might come up at his planned meeting with the Prime Minister. His team was not encouraging:

> It was noted that if his [Enthoven's] ideas were to be implemented in full, this would be likely to lead away from the move towards equality

of access to hospitals, and reintroduce the pre-1948 situation under which quite extensive travelling had often been required by those living away from the major teaching hospitals. All the evidence was that both DHAs, patients and GPs preferred locally based services, except for the treatment of rare forms of disease where this might not be the best solution. Districts could already 'buy-in' services, and it was highly desirable to continue to promote information which would allow patients to weigh up the advantage of quicker treatment against the disadvantages of being further from home. Enthoven had correctly identified a fourfold variance in the rate of referral by GPs, for which there was no obvious explanation in terms of pattern of sickness. Both Enthoven's proposals and those of the Department of Health were intended to meet a common end, namely the efficient use of resources. Both accepted the need for a more information driven system. It was, however, important to deliver on the basis of agreed programmes rather diverting too much attention to the study of alternative models.[70]

That was the end of that, or so they thought!

Throughout this early period, attempts were being made to sort out the boundary between policy and management. This was a tough philosophical challenge, and empires were also at risk. During February and March a series of meetings had been held to see if a sensible accommodation could be found. Paige wanted to know what the boundary was between the Management Board and the Health and Personal Social Services (HPSS) Policy Group, and to get a feel for the boundary's permeability.[71]

Chris France, who was at this stage the civil servant in charge of the Policy Group, put the issue in context:

> It goes without saying that the Policy Group does not seek to do its business in an ivory tower. It is right that there should be two-way consultation between the Policy Board and the Management Board in relation to policy issues. The Management Board can and should point out to us problems which our policies can present for management, and the Policy Group would certainly expect to have regard to them and to modify proposals accordingly. The need for an adequate working relationship will persist wherever one cuts the robe.[71]

The various Policy Divisions were asked to indicate on a four-point scale where they would place the Management Board's interest in their major tasks. The results were as follows:

- *very strong:* 24 – including hospital services, maternity, children, catering and domestic services and private health
- *strong:* 10 – including Public Health Laboratories, overseas visitors, ethnic health, rehabilitation, primary healthcare and CHCs
- *weak:* 31 – including unorthodox medicine, voluntary work, abortion, family planning, sexually transmitted diseases and complaints
- *none:* 24 – including confidentiality of patient records, ethical matters, child abuse, food hygiene, nutrition, smoking and children in care.

In March 1985 Stowe intervened:

> There are volumes of history on how best to operate the operational and policy functions in respect of health authorities. The only principle that matters is that all officials have a single accountability to the Secretary of State. There are no representatives of the NHS in the Department. The objective of Griffiths was to permit a high-ranking official to give all his time to the management of health authorities, supported by others who were similarly dedicated, without being preoccupied as I and others were with policy issues.[71]

A month later Stowe convened a top-of-the-office meeting to resolve the matter. It was agreed that a neat division between policy and management was not possible. They needed to work in harmony. Everyone was exhorted to pull together, but beneath the surface the arguments continued, for in the minds of some officials there was a clear distinction between managing the NHS and taking forward health policy.

The bureaucracy at the centre was now very complex indeed. There were twice-monthly NHS Management Board meetings scheduled, meetings with regional general managers, and joint Management Board and regional general manager meetings. There were meetings with regional chairmen, some of which involved ministers. All of this was on top of the internal meeting structures of the Department of Health.

In August 1985, Paige met the University Hospitals Association, which complained about university cuts and the Department's revenue allocation policy (RAWP). This policy, which was designed to secure a more equitable distribution of revenue funds between the English regions, was hitting London and the South-East particularly hard. The University Hospitals Association told him how much they resented their loss of direct access to the DHSS. The district health authorities, to whom they were now accountable, were considered too responsive to political interference.[72] They wanted to go back to an earlier age. Paige listened but made no comment. However, this issue was to resurface a few years later as ideas about trusts developed.

The table overleaf shows an analysis of NHS Management Board business from 1 April 1985 for one year, and is taken from minutes of the meetings. Where minutes are missing, agendas have been used where these were available.[73–81] The period covers the second year of the analysis of business for the Supervisory Board.

An early judgement

While the Management Board was picking up steam, Stowe was already thinking about the next election and ruminating about the future. He prepared a personal note for Fowler on 4 June 1985 scanning the future policy territory so that ideas for a new Parliament could be developed.[57] The scan was very wide indeed, but included a section on the management of the NHS. A copy was passed to Paige by a friendly civil servant a couple of weeks later. Paige got one of his staff to make a handwritten copy, and prepared an immediate response.[57] He was very angry.

Topic discussed	Number of the meeting in which it was discussed*
Board's role and procedures	3, 6, 7, 10, 19, 21
Regional chairmen	5, 7, 8, 13
Regional general manager roles	7, 8, 9
Short-term programmes	3, 4, 8, 9, 16, 20
Cost improvements and productivity	3, 4
Public expenditure on NHS	14
Management Accounting Framework and budgeting	4, 7, 8
Competitive tendering	6, 8, 10
Resource allocation and RAWP	12, 21
Development of performance review system	12, 15, 21
NHS performance indicators	12, 21
85 objectives	4
Matters concerning individual Regions	4, 5, 10, 11, 13, 15, 17, 18, 19
Medical manpower	8, 10, 12, 14
Non-medical manpower	3, 8, 16, 21
Pay review body/Whitley matters	7, 8, 12, 13, 19, 21
Property and works, estates	4, 7, 8, 20
Procurement and supplies	4, 7
Non-ambulance transport scrutiny	5
Ambulance service	5, 10
Validation of waiting lists	5, 21
Communications, including traffic survey	3, 4, 6, 7, 8, 10, 21
National guidelines to RHAs	13
AIDS	13, 14
Körner Report on Information	7, 8, 12, 14
Research matters	7, 8, 11, 16
Nursing topics, including education and training	5, 6, 8, 11, 14, 17, 20, 21
Private practice in NHS hospitals	8, 9, 10, 16
Medical errors	8
Energy conservation	11
Unit general managers	11, 19
Crown immunity	12, 19
Enthoven Report	9
Supra-regional services	14, 17
Community Child Health Services	14
Artificial Limb and Appliances Centres	15, 16, 19, 20, 21
Community medicine	15, 20
Ethnic minorities	16
Presentation to Prime Minister	10, 19
Violence in hospitals	19
Quality assurance structures	20
Financial management	20
Stanley Royd Inquiry into food poisoning	21
Legionnaires' disease	21

* Meetings 1 and 2 are not included as they were classed as interim meetings.

In the note Stowe had concluded that the Health Services Supervisory Board (HSSB), which by this stage had been operating for 18 months, was showing few signs of being a success. All of the key policy issues in his view were much wider than the NHS. He would prefer to move to a Health and Social Services Board that would in its membership 'steer away from management towards eminence in a professional field or a broader-based independence.'

> In any case, the Supervisory Board had always been the weakest point in the Griffiths Report because it was primarily designed to keep ministers and permanent secretaries out of the Management Board. Since ministers and their permanent secretaries were wholly in favour of the Management Board, and had a hand in devising it, this was an unnecessary device.[57]

> It was [Stowe stated] defective in that:

> - The powers of the Secretary of State cannot be put into commission, so the Board concept here is not only especially unreal, but misleading: it cannot be more than any group of advisers sitting around the Secretary of State's table.
> - Even so, as a formal group of advisers it is a strange mixture of ministers and some – but not the most relevant – officials, with one outsider.
> - In consequence it has tended to focus on NHS management questions.[57]

In relation to the Management Board, Stowe pointed up the tensions with both ministers and the regional chairmen. It was not just Department of Health ministers who were involved, but also the Treasury and Downing Street when questions of pay and NHS investment came up for discussion. Stowe thought that there was a natural tendency (encouraged by the NHS) for the Board to pull away, both physically and politically, from ministers. 'But,' as he explained, 'ministers could not abdicate their responsibilities.'[57]

Six months in and there was little progress to report other than what was already in the pipeline. The Management Board would in his view have to start delivering soon by leaning on health authorities, and as it did ministers would be drawn in.

Stowe was very direct with Fowler in this note. The Management Board would need Fowler's support if it came under challenge by recalcitrant health authorities. As he put it:

> The whole edifice rests at present on the Secretary of State's powers of direction. The Board itself is an administrative device and no more (or less) authoritative than any other collection of civil servants. Although we have pulled off a neat trick by setting it up quickly without legislation, there is a question about whether it can last.[57]

The Board, as it then existed, was in his view 'little more than a useful engine to establish the credibility of general management until after the next election.'[57]

Stowe had even worked out what stage two might look like in order to eliminate an administrative tier, reduce bureaucracy and establish a clear line of control and accountability from the unit to the centre. It involved converting the Management Board into a special health authority.

Stowe's second stage of development

1 The NHSMB would be set up as a special health authority under existing powers as the Central Health Authority for England (CHAE). It could retain the title NHSMB if desired.
2 It would have a full-time chairman (Paige) and a full-time chief executive (perhaps Fairey). Its members would, at least transitionally, include four or five of the best regional chairmen.
3 Its staff would be drawn from the NHS and the Department of Health, but they would be NHS employees, not civil servants. There would be a reduction in the size of the Department of Health.
4 RHAs would be abolished as authorities, and this would require legislation.
5 Their functions would be transferred either to CHAE (e.g. strategic planning) or to designated district authorities (e.g. ambulances).
6 Bodies such as the Supply Council and the NHS Training Authority would disappear into CHAE.
7 DHAs would be accountable to CHAE.

Don Wilson, the chairman of the Mersey Region, was even pencilled in as a possible successor to Victor Paige once Paige had retired.

This was explosive thinking only six months into the new structures, and Paige reacted quickly and strongly with a handwritten note to Stowe on 13 June 1985:

> To contemplate such prospects – even when the present Board is still incomplete and has been operating for but a few weeks in a diminished form – reveals a much lesser commitment to the sanctity of the earlier conclusions than I had ever envisaged.[57]

Paige is referring here to the arguments that were advanced during the discussions leading to his appointment about the difficulties of separating the Management Board from the Department of Health, and the fact that the NHS could not cope with yet another reorganisation. If such a change was contemplated within the next two or three years, then in his view 'it was relevant to both the way the Board set out on its journey and the destination it planned to reach'.

Although Paige acknowledged the tensions referred to by Stowe, he argued that time would ease them. He demanded the right to be present when these ideas were discussed with Norman Fowler. If he was not, his position 'would become a mockery.'[57]

A meeting with Fowler followed, during which Paige rehearsed the by now familiar arguments. For his new Board to work, he argued, it must have well-defined accountability and authority. 'I recognise absolutely the ultimate authority of the Secretary of State and ministers, but beneath that is a complex matrix. I do not believe we are yet clear about it; certainly I am not.'[56]

Paige then posed a series of questions to illustrate the dilemma.

Who he asked [ministers/Supervisory Board/Management Board/Permanent Secretary/CMO or regional chairmen] initiates policy thinking, recommends action, decides to proceed and implements policy in the following areas:

- major health policies and priorities (transplants, hips, aids)
- financing of community care
- bids to the Treasury for funding (Public Expenditure Survey Committee round)
- health implications of Social Security initiatives
- NHS Corporate Plan
- pay structures and policies
- hospital consultants' contracts?

Paige obtained no clear answers except that, at the end of the day, everything ended up with the Secretary of State. Fowler took no immediate action with regard to Stowe's paper.

Paige's relationships with the regional chairmen had been reasonably good at a personal level, although there had been an early disagreement about the decision to appoint Peach as chairman of the NHS Training Authority. As Peach puts it, 'they felt they should have been approached to get their opinion before the decision was made.'[82] The chairmen were determined as a group to maintain their direct link to the Secretary of State as promised by Fowler in 1983.[44] In April 1985 they had dinner with Stowe and followed up the discussion with a letter drafted by Sir Peter Baldwin, the chairman of the SE Thames Region and a former Permanent Secretary at the Department of Transport.[83]

They restated how much they 'cherished the direct relationship they had with the Secretary of State, to whom of course they were directly and personably accountable'. They acknowledged that the Management Board would want to monitor *their* officers but also wanted the Board to focus on policy development and improving healthcare. They wanted all consultation with experts within the NHS (treasurers, medical officers and personnel officers) to be channelled through them and the inter-regional secretariat that they had created. They wanted to keep their hands on the reins of power. Stowe was of the view, from quite early days, that the regional chairmen, by virtue of the process for appointing them, had to be regarded as part of the political rather than the managerial system, and because of this, ministers would never agree to break the direct link to themselves.[2]

There was a hefty programme of change to management systems and practice in the NHS. General managers were to be appointed throughout the system with performance-based contracts. New management structures had to be introduced (within a framework of strict management costs and a philosophy of decentralisation) and performance review systems established with the new and much vaunted performance indicators. There was a daunting programme of work in the personnel and industrial relations field. A long-term pay strategy was needed, as were better manpower planning and financial control. Ian Mills, the new Director of Finance, had quickly concluded that unless the doctors were involved in the management of budgets, they had little or no incentive to control costs. He launched the Resource Management Initiative in 1986 at six pilot sites in

England. Its aim was to establish the effect on the quality and quantity of patient care when clinicians were fully involved in the management of their hospitals, supported by information from computerised databases on the resources used to treat individual patients. This programme was later to be rolled out across the NHS as one of the key elements of the internal market.[75]

On 22 July 1985 the Prime Minister, Margaret Thatcher, held a meeting to discuss progress. She urged Paige and his new Board to 'approach their task with vigour. It should be apparent to all that the NHS was under new management'. She said that 'The Board should seek radical solutions and if necessary seek reinforcement from the private sector.' She asked 'Was there enough training?'[71]

She particularly wanted Paige and his Board to pursue improvements in performance as vigorously as possible. The same meeting agreed that the Board would produce an annual report (with a 'popular' version) and review consultant contracts. Mrs Thatcher took a very close interest in the development of performance indicators and pay policy. When asked to pick a health authority at random to demonstrate the new computer model, she disconcertingly chose Newcastle rather than her own constituency of Barnet. She was by all accounts impressed. Earlier in the same meeting she had given everyone, including her ministers, a hard time for building in an assumption that future pay would be broadly in line with inflation. At her insistence, the next set of NHS budget projections assumed a figure lower than inflation.[57]

However, underneath the flurry of activity some basic unanswered questions began to re-emerge.

In November 1985 Stowe wrote to his senior colleagues:

> The Secretary of State reacted (privately, to me) very sharply recently when he saw papers saying that a Management Board had decided something. The Secretary of State is concerned – and rightly – that ministers' position and authority are not undermined. I think we all understand the rules of the game, and I hope all three management boards (the Department Management Board, the NHS Management Board and the Social Security Management Board) will be sensitive to them. We have to take the trick of operating with authority without usurping it.[57]

Paige reacted strongly, arguing that in serving the Secretary of State the Management Board must take decisions. If Norman Fowler had problems with the actions of the Management Board he should say so. The use of the word 'decide' was dropped in future minutes of the Management Board.

Len Peach had joined Paige in November 1985 as Director of Personnel, seconded from IBM. He 'took the Griffiths Report as his Bible' and began to build his own team. It was slow going, and even getting a secretary proved to be a challenge. Every new post had to be defined, graded and argued about. It took Peach six months to recruit a communications manager. He was philosophical about the delays – he was now in the Civil Service rather than in industry.[82]

Paige, on the other hand, found that his patience was wearing very thin. The reappointment of regional chairmen had been up for review, and his advice had been sought. He consulted his colleagues and concluded that two of the older chairmen, both aged over 70 years, should be replaced together with a third who was widely regarded as being out of his depth. In Paige's view, setting and maintaining standards started at the top. He saw these chairmen, who were part time, as having a crucial executive role. The rest of the Department did not see them in this way, and treated them more as on-the-ground political advisers. Paige's advice was ignored and all three individuals were reappointed. As he expressed it to Stowe at the time, 'mediocrity won.'[62]

By this time the negotiations about general managers' contracts and pay had still not been settled and were approaching what he regarded as a 'tatty compromise'. He had wanted a bold new imaginative message shaped around management contracts and pay. What was close to agreement would, he thought, 'switch people off.' Once again the effective management of the NHS was, in his view, to take a subordinate position to other problems and the service would console itself with 'better than nothing.'[62]

Paige did not regard either of these issues as fundamental, but they fuelled his growing anxieties about management credibility and integrity. He wrote a personal note to Stowe: 'If one is not vigilant, easy compromise can become a habit, addictive, a way of life. That can lead to awfully weak management. No thank you.'[57]

However, Stowe was under pressure from the politicians, and one minister in particular had complained strongly that Paige had to learn to act as a Permanent Secretary.[2]

By Easter, Paige had had enough and decided it was time to go. He sent a handwritten note to Stowe: 'Sorry, but Thursday reopened my anxieties about the future. As you know they were very close to the surface. So I think we are discussing how and when and not if. We should probably act sooner rather than later.'[57]

His resignation was announced on 3 June 1986, to the surprise of his colleagues on the Management Board, most of whom got only a few hours' notice. One in particular felt slightly betrayed by Paige: they 'had been brought into this with Victor as the leader.'[82]

In his letter of resignation, Paige reiterated his belief in the value of general management in the NHS and pointed up the tension between managerial and political perspectives: 'Ministers and the Chairman of the Management Board can approach the same issue with different perspectives, priorities, objectives and restraints.'[57]

The Guardian announced that his departure was a blow to the top management structure of the DHSS. *The Financial Times* presented it as a long-running disagreement with Norman Fowler over the right to manage the NHS. The tabloids blamed the civil servants. According to *The Mail*, 'Whitehall defeats Mr Efficiency', when Paige admitted that the burden of coping with civil servants and a working environment more akin to *Yes Minister* than the board-room had proved too much.

Fowler's reply acknowledged that 'things had not worked out'. In his memoirs Fowler is more forthcoming, and in regretting Paige's decision to resign he acknowledged:

> He had a point. When Victor Paige became the first general manager of the Health Service he found himself in a very different job from any that he or anyone else had occupied before. He was not the chief

executive of a big corporation but in an uneasy no man's land between the Department of Health and the service.[84]

'However,' Fowler would also argue, 'as the minister's general manager you have quite a lot of power. It depends how you use it and it depends on your ability to use it. But it is not easy.' He later reflected, 'We needed an exceptional half-politician, half-manager.'[29]

Kenneth Clarke also wrote a personal letter to Paige expressing both his regret and his mystification about what went wrong:

> I am sorry that it all came to this sad end, and I feel a little guilty about my part in talking you into the job. However, I am sure you feel that you did achieve a very great deal during your time at the Management Board.[85]

Stowe regarded his inability to persuade Paige not to resign as a 'dismal memory', for he believed that 'We understood each other. We were not aristocrats, we didn't come from the upper-middle-class gentry'. In his view Paige had achieved much in a short time.[2]

Stowe and Paige met at the Athenaeum Club shortly after the resignation. Stowe asked for Paige's advice about the next steps.

> I gave my reply. With the present structure there is only one answer. The chairman of the Management Board if it is to be continued has to be a minister.[62]

Paige said little at the time about his experience as chairman, and resisted the press clamour for comment. He left quietly and with dignity. He did not seek a meeting with Mrs Thatcher, although Fowler would have gone with him.[29] He wanted to avoid a heavy slanging match and damage to the credibility of the Secretary of State.[86] However, he did give evidence to two Select Committees once the dust had settled and his successor had been appointed.

The first appearance was in April 1987, before the Social Services Committee.[87] He confirmed his continued support for the introduction of general management into the NHS itself, but thought that Griffiths had got it wrong with regard to the central management of the NHS inside the Department of Health and Social Security. The intention (if there had ever been one) to devolve executive accountability and authority from the Secretary of State was never realised. He explained, 'Ministers take all the important decisions – political, strategic and managerial.' The Management Board could only advise and influence ministers and 'did not manage in the way that would be understood in industry and commerce.' As Chairman of the Management Board, he and his colleagues 'served, not decided.'[57] The Management Board advised, but did not manage.

His second appearance came a year later in May 1988 when he was invited to give evidence to the Treasury and Civil Service Committee about the relevance of Next Steps Agencies to the health sector.

The Next Steps Programme was the brainchild of the Downing Street Efficiency Unit, led by Robin Ibbs. The plan, which had been presented to Margaret Thatcher in May 1987, was for discrete parts of the government machine to be hived off into semi-autonomous agencies (e.g. the Benefits Agency or the Meteorological Office). They remained accountable to ministers but would operate with relative freedom within clear performance targets. Ibbs also wanted a change in the British constitution, by law if necessary, 'to quash the fiction that ministers can be genuinely responsible for everything done by officials in their name.' In the event this proved too much for the Treasury, who persuaded Mrs Thatcher not to go that far. They also insisted it was essential that they continued to be involved in the control of budgets, manpower and national pay negotiations.[88] By 1998 there were 140 agencies, including a few (such as the Serious Crime Squad) which operated along Next Steps lines. The idea had gone further than most imagined it would in 1987.

Paige used the opportunity to return to the theme he had developed in his first appearance of an independent corporation to run the NHS. In his judgement such an organisation would lead to 'the NHS being better managed than at present, would give better value for public money, and provide a better health service for our people'. He said that an essential component of a step forward such as this 'would be to resolve the problems created by a muddled and complex chain of command.' He understood the political difficulties associated with such a proposal, but thought that 'fertile minds' could find a solution.[89]

His advice had little impact, and the NHS played no real part in the Next Steps Programme.

With the benefit of hindsight, Fowler now takes a similar view to Paige:

> Here you had the Health Service and here the Department of Health which was full of advisers. The Health Service was being managed out there and it seems to me that the sensible way of actually doing this, which would have met Victor's point, was that we should have set up a Health Service Commission, a separate entity, financed from public funds. Under this model the final accountability of the Secretary of State would remain, but the Commission would manage the NHS on his behalf.[29]

In retrospect, nearly 20 years after his short appointment as Chief Executive, Paige reflects as follows:

> Looking back it was a fascinating experience, but I should never have accepted the appointment. The Griffith Report was interesting but massively flawed. I was put under a lot of pressure to accept the appointment but I really should have rejected it. It was and should have been an enormous challenge, which I would have welcomed. But it wasn't. It was doomed to failure. They should not have been looking for a manager. It was really best suited to a highly imaginative administrator.[57]

So was Paige sold a bogus prospectus? The advertisement for the job says that the Chairman 'will report direct to the Secretary of State and will carry principal responsibility for the discharge of the Secretary of State's powers relating to the management of the NHS.' It is clear that Stowe, at least, made it plain that this did not mean managing the NHS, and that decision making could not, and would not, be devolved by ministers. As Stowe was to explain much later in 2001:

> Beginning with Victor Paige and ending with Nigel Crisp, you have been up hill and down dale trying to sort out this division of

responsibilities between ministers and Permanent Secretary and something called the Management Board which has got outsiders on it. But
in fact they are outsiders exercising the minister's powers only for as
long as the minister says you can have my powers to play with. The
moment he says 'you can't', you can't, and that was the story of Victor
Paige, which ended in tears.[2]

Stowe had grown up in a system where he wielded very substantial personal
authority, but always in the name of his political masters.

Others, including it seems the Prime Minister, the public and NHS management, thought that Paige had indeed been brought in to sort out the NHS, to
exercise strong leadership and to make decisions in operational areas devolved to
him by the Secretary of State. His leadership style was to be modelled on industry,
not on the Civil Service. Paige demanded clarity; the system offered subtlety. The
image and the reality never matched.

Chapter 3

Timeline

1986

June

- Len Peach was appointed as acting Chairman of the NHS Management Board. A meeting was convened at Hurlingham Club by Norman Fowler to discuss and sort out political and policy priorities.

July

- Len Peach met Margaret Thatcher.

September

- Mrs Thatcher invited the regional chairmen and managers for dinner at Number 10.

October

- The Cumberlege Report, *Neighbourhood Nursing: a focus for care*,[90] was published. This was a report on the community nursing teams for England.

November

- The Minister of State, Tony Newton, became Chairman of the Management Board, with Sir Roy Griffiths as Vice-Chairman.
- Len Peach was appointed as Chief Executive and retained his role as Director of Personnel.

1987

January

- There was growing concern in London about the spread of AIDS.
- *Towards a Better Healthcare: a case for change*,[57] a strictly confidential paper, was produced by Kenneth Stowe and the policy team for ministers.
- Mrs Thatcher held a meeting to discuss future health policy.

March

- The last meeting of the Health Services Supervisory Board was held.

April

- Victor Paige appeared before the Social Services Committee of the House of Commons.

May

- The Next Steps Programme was presented to Mrs Thatcher by Robin Ibbs.

June

- The Conservatives returned at the General Election. John Moore was appointed as Secretary of State, and Nicholas Scott and Tony Newton as Ministers of Health.
- Newton remained as Chairman of the Management Board.

October

- Great storm hit southern England.
- The regional chairmen warned ministers of the growing financial crisis.
- Black Monday in the City.
- The Birmingham Children's Hospital crisis hit the headlines.
- *Achieving a Balance*[92] was published, outlining a policy that was designed to create a better career structure for hospital doctors.

December

- The Presidents of the medical Royal Colleges issued a press release about the financial crisis in the NHS.
- John Moore became ill and Tony Newton stood in for him.

1988

January

- Sir Kenneth Stowe retired and Christopher France became Permanent Secretary at the Department of Health.
- The Acheson Report[93] on public health was published.
- The Presidents of the medical Royal Colleges met John Moore to demand a greater investment in the NHS.
- Mrs Thatcher announced a review of the NHS on the TV programme *Panorama*.

March

- The Griffiths Report, *Community Care: agenda for action*,[36] was published.
- *Improving Management in Government: the next steps*[88] was published by the Cabinet Efficiency Unit.
- Paige gave evidence to the Treasury and Social Services Committee.

April

- The Family Practitioner Committees became Family Health Service Authorities accountable to regional health authorities.

July

- The DHSS was split into two. Kenneth Clarke became Secretary of State for Health and David Mellor became Minister of Health.
- John Moore took over Social Security.

December

- Edwina Currie resigned during the egg controversy.

1989

January

- The White Paper *Working for Patients: the Health Service caring for the 1990s*[94] was launched with a series of teleconferences. It proposed the creation of what became known as the 'internal market'.
- Len Peach returned to IBM, and Duncan Nichol took over as Chief Executive.

April

- The Department of Health published *A Strategy for Nursing*.[95]

May

- The Health Services Supervisory Board was replaced by the Policy Board.
- The Management Board became the NHS Management Executive, chaired by the Chief Executive, Duncan Nichol, and not by a Minister.
- Kenneth Stowe published his book *On Caring for the National Health*,[96] and recalled that 'Griffiths' was nearly a disaster.

Len Peach, 1986–89

With Paige's sudden departure, much thought had to be given to the next steps. Len Peach was asked to take on the role as acting chairman until such time as decisions could be made about the future. He was an interesting choice. The deputy chairman was Graham Hart, but he was a civil servant and making him chairman would not fit with the business image that the DHSS was still promoting. Peach came from industry and did fit the image.

The discussions continued throughout the summer months and focused again on accountability. In July, Stowe briefed the Secretary of State for a meeting with the Prime Minister: 'The resignation of Paige illustrates a problem of introducing a managerial administrative framework into a national framework for which ministers are accountable to Parliament.'[71]

The same paper again rehearsed the options for change as follows.

- Abolish the Management Board.
- Maintain it in a non-statutory form.
- Set up a statutory health authority under the 1977 Act.
- Set up a statutory authority with executive responsibilities and a power to direct health authorities in England.
- Set up an independent National Health Corporation.

The Select Committee of the House of Commons also had a view, and made it plain that they would oppose any move that diminished the direct accountability of ministers to Parliament for the NHS. Barney Heyhoe MP insisted that Members of Parliament attached considerable importance to their ability to raise, with the minister of the day, issues affecting the healthcare of their constituents both as groups and as individuals. They recommended that before seeking a successor to Paige, ministers should agree with them what the responsibilities of the NHS Management Board and its chairman were, including the Board chairman's relationship with regional chairmen.[97]

In November 1986 it was announced that the Minister of State for Health, Tony Newton, would take on the role of chairman of the Management Board. Roy Griffiths would be vice-chairman and Len Peach was appointed as chief executive.

Lord Tony Newton

Tony Newton was born in 1937 and went to Oxford University, where he played a predominant role in university politics, and became President of the Union. He joined the Conservative Party Research Department before being elected as an MP for Braintree, Essex from 1974 to 1997. He was Health Minister and Chairman of the Management Board in the Conservative Government from 1986 to 1988, Secretary of State for Social Security from 1989 to 1992, and Lord President of the Council and Leader of the House of Commons from 1992 to 1997. He was appointed Chairman of the Northeast Essex Mental Health NHS Trust in 2001. He has also chaired the

West London Health Partnership Forum. He is Chairman of the Council on Tribunals.

Sir Len Peach, Chief Executive of the NHS, 1986–89[82]

Len Peach was born in Walsall, Staffordshire in 1932, the eldest of five children. A scholarship to the grammar school allowed him to do school certificate and A-levels. He did his national service as a Second Lieutenant in the Infantry, and served in the Suez Canal Zone. Later, in 1953, he read history at Pembroke College, Oxford.

After working for Randolph Churchill for six months researching a book on the life of Lord Derby, Peach decided that he did not want to become an academic, and successfully applied to John Thompson's of Wolverhampton, a nuclear engineering works. They ran a scheme that allowed arts graduates to gain engineering experience, and he spent a year mostly on the shop floor. Thompson's, on deciding that they needed a personnel officer, asked him to attend the London School of Economics for a year to do a diploma. He passed with distinction.

He returned to Thompson's, where he stayed only a short time as his interest in personnel management was growing. He joined the West Midlands Gas Board at a time when nationalised industries were doing well in terms of personnel management, and here he ran management quality courses. His next move was to set up a training system at Solihull College of Further Education. At the age of 29 years he joined IBM as Assistant Management Development Co-ordinator, and remained with them for many years. During his career he was Personnel Manager of the Greenock plant, Director of Personnel for the UK, Director of Personnel for Europe, and from 1975 Head of Personnel and Corporate Affairs in the UK.

He held the position of Vice-President of the Institute of Personnel Managers from 1979 to 1982 and of President from 1982 to 1985.

In November 1985, Peach was seconded to the Department of Health as the Director of Personnel. From June 1986 until November 1986 he became temporary chairman of the NHS Management Board, and was appointed Chief Executive in November 1986. He combined this post with that of Director of Personnel. He resigned in order to return to IBM in January 1989, but continued with the NHS Training Authority until 1991–92. On retiring from IBM in 1992 he became Chairman of the Police Complaints Authority and later Commissioner for Public Appointments.

This was, according to the *NHS Management Bulletin*, the strongest team to lead health authority management that the Government had ever put together.[98]

In Stowe's view this new arrangement for the Management Board had a number of merits. It reflected an agreed view that immediate past frustrations had not undermined the case for a management board at the centre: 'It was not to be a body to manage in a line manager sense but to conduct efficiently those functions relating to the management of health authorities that had to be performed at the centre.'[96]

Norman Fowler's report to the Supervisory Board on 3 November 1986 was more direct: 'The changes have been made in order to remove any appearance of a division of authority between ministers and the Board.'[99]

The changes were introduced with a minimum of controversy. The iron grip of parliamentary accountability had won again. Not everyone was convinced that it was the right answer, and some continued to argue the case for a Director General accountable to the Secretary of State but outside the Department of Health.[100]

To get the job of chief executive, Peach had gone through a Civil Service interview process with little difficulty, although there was a senior Civil Service candidate. Peach came from a personnel management rather than a chief executive background and had, in Stowe's judgement, a flair for multi-disciplinary management.[2] He was happy to play a role in a large and complex team, and he would not demand the clarity with regard to personal powers and accountability that Paige had sought.

This did not stop him making decisions in appropriate areas, but to use his own words 'My whole experience was indirect power. I never had a job in which I had direct power, but I believed I exercised a lot of influence by mechanisms and professionalism.'[82]

He combined his role of chief executive with that of director of personnel, and this shaped much of his contribution to the Board. Rolling out performance assessment and performance-related pay was in his judgement crucial to the successful implementation of the Griffiths reforms. He regarded his chairmanship of the NHS Training Authority as particularly important, and he planned to transform the organisation into a major engine for change. He did not seek or have any responsibility for health policy or the oversight of the Family Practitioner Services. He saw himself 'as the Chief Operating Officer of the NHS.' He never saw himself in a strategic role 'because he had never applied for a job in a strategic role.'[82]

The membership of the Management Board at this stage was as follows.

Chairman, Minister of Health	Tony Newton
Vice-Chairman	Roy Griffiths
Chief Executive and Director of Personnel	Len Peach
Director of Health Authority Finance	John James
Director of Planning and Information Technology	Michael Fairey
Director of Operations (Personnel)	Peter Wormald
Director of Health Authority Liaison	Anthony Merifield
Director of Operations	Graham Hart, followed by Mike Malone-Lee in 1987
Director of Financial Management	Ian Mills
Chief Medical Officer	Donald Acheson
Chief Nursing Officer	Anne Poole
Director of NHS Distribution and Procurement	Tom Critchley
Non-Executive Director	Duncan Nichol
Property Adviser	Idris Pearce

Far from resenting the fact that a minister was taking over the chairmanship of the Management Board, Peach welcomed it: 'it meant you could talk policy at the Management Board.'[82] Duncan Nichol continued as a non-executive member. He regarded himself as a part-time member with an operational perspective. He was not a representative of the regions and did not report back to them, but he did act as a valuable linkage point. Regional managers did attend the Board on occasion, but were treated with caution as outsiders. Brian Edwards, RGM Trent, made a presentation to the Board on quality initiatives in his region in June 1988. Peach had to specifically agree that, as an outsider, he could stay for the discussion following his presentation.

Tony Newton did not have a reputation as a good chairman, but was respected as a pleasant and intelligent minister. Edwina Currie, his colleague at the time, expressed it thus: 'Tony Newton is a sad case. Now in his sixth year at the DHSS and really fed up with it. Did all Norman Fowler's legwork for years and got no thanks or reward. But he is disorganised and poor at taking decisions.'[101]

On 9 and 10 June 1986, Fowler convened a special two-day meeting at the Hurlingham Club in London.[102] The aim was 'to enable ministers to identify what they saw as the political priorities on the first day, and on the second day how best to carry forward a programme of action.' Ministers were joined by Peach, the Chief Medical Officer, the Chief Nursing Officer, Hart, Fairey and others when they presented papers. There were papers on medical education, medicines, community care, elderly people, primary healthcare, staffing, medical developments, private sector healthcare, resource allocation, Inner London, NHS estate, waiting lists, prevention policies, mental health and finance. The outcomes of the conference shaped the Department's policy agenda for some time into the future, and much of it fell outside the remit of the Management Board.

The discussions about primary care led to the identification of a number of initiatives that could proceed without waiting for the outcome of negotiations with the BMA on the major review. These included practice leaflets, pilot neighbourhood nursing schemes and local quality control teams. However, Fowler did not want to push the role of the private sector in primary care. The proposed Green Paper on community care was aired. Medicines management got a good run as ministers continued the search for economies in the drug budget. They wondered about economic incentives to appropriate prescribing for GPs, and they agreed on a pilot public information campaign. Waiting lists were discussed in some detail, and Fowler asked for plans to be drawn up for a full-blooded campaign to get them reduced in 1987–88. A clear plan of action on health promotion was to be prepared.

A discussion about Labour Party plans for directly elected members of health authorities (which ministers rejected as unworkable) led into another discussion about accountability and independent corporations. Fowler wanted another look at the alternative methods of funding the NHS. He judged that the time was not right for the introduction of health insurance, but thought that increased charges were worth looking at, together with the possible privatisation of ophthalmic and dental services. There was a lot of interest in this conference, including some from the National Audit Office, who asked for a set of papers. They were rebuffed on the grounds that the event had been little more than a brainstorming session for ministers.

In the midst of all this high policy, Peach got on with sorting out what he regarded as the basics. In addition to the contract and pay issues, he was very concerned to improve communication systems within the NHS and to improve information flows. This meant implementing the Körner Report[23] on health service information.

He was also drawn to a clutch of nursing problems. These included discussions about the implementation of the Cumberlege Report on community nursing,[90] the reform of nurse training (Project 2000) and the new nurse grading system. This grading system was later to cause many problems when individual nurses appealed against the grade that they had been allocated.

In medicine, *Achieving a Balance*[92] was launched, which was designed to reduce junior doctors' hours of work and at the same time ensure that all doctors in training had the opportunity to become a consultant or general practitioner. This was to be a long drawn-out agony as junior doctor posts were slowly reallocated around the country.

But behind all of this was a deeper problem that had its roots in the return to full employment and the career choices of young people. A paper prepared for the cancelled Health Service Supervisory Board meeting in April 1987 puts it succinctly:

> The service currently recruits about 30% of female school leavers with between 5 'O'- and 2 'A'-levels. This pool is projected to decline by 27% between 1982 and 1992 whilst the NHS plan shows a manpower growth of 6%.[103]

Peach would have liked to start an NHS Staff College along the lines of the Civil Service model. Why should the Civil Service have a staff college for 120 000 people? It was because, he argued, it was important to their culture. So why not have one for an organisation with a million staff and 10 000 managers?[82] He received little support from senior managers in the NHS, who did not take well to the idea of management education for the NHS being run from the centre. They preferred more local arrangements.

A review of Management Board business in the second half of 1987 shows a clear focus on financial and manpower issues. The table opposite shows an analysis of Management Board business each month from June 1987 to March 1988.[104] Roy Griffiths took the chair on the occasions when the Minister could not attend.

The Health Service Supervisory Board had continued to meet throughout this period. It received a regular update from the Management Board, which always dominated its business, but the Supervisory Board did play a significant role in policy development. It discussed community medicine, AIDS, the consumer, housing and health, and NHS procurement. Occasionally it had extended debates about clinical areas such as genetics, mental health or services for the disabled. The membership had changed in 1986 with the addition of Sir Raymond Hoffenberg, the President of the Royal College of Physicians, in February 1986, and Sir Donald Wilson, Regional Chairman for the Mersey Region, in 1987. It was never the powerhouse of the DHSS, but Fowler in particular valued it as a sounding board. He was also conscious that it would not do any harm to let the NHS see that the Board had a leading physician and a regional chairman among its membership.

Business	22/6	20/7	3/8	14/9	5/10	19/10	2/11	16/11	18/11	i/2	15/2	7/3	21/3
Waiting lists	+	+											
Pay	+		+										
Cash limits	+	+			+	+							+
PESC	+						+						
Medical manpower	+												
General manpower	+										+		
Nurse staffing and training	+	+						+	+		+		
Communications		+		+									
Acute sector trends			+										
Overseas doctors			+										
Health promotion													
Administration and clerical staffing				+									
Quality management				+									
Senior managers' pay				+									
Competitive tendering					+	+							
Evidence to Select Committee					+	+							
Night nursing						+							
Cervical cancer							+						
RAWP							+						
Strategic planning								+			+		
Aims and objectives								+					
Directors' reports									+				
Industrial relations									+	+	+	+	+
Birmingham Children's Hospital									+				
Consultant contracts									+				
NHS Review													
NHS Supplies										+			
Resource management													
Regional chairmen													+

However, the reality was that ministers themselves had opinions about and attitudes to health policy that usually dominated the decision-making process. For example, Edwina Currie recalls in her diary for 31 August 1987:

> Visit to Gravesend tomorrow; they're proposing a complicated re-organisation of local health services and we are being bounced into it. In the long run the Health Authority wants a huge £60 million hospital, all on one site but I'm against that – inhuman, cold, unattractive and fiendishly expensive.[101]

The financial crisis and the Thatcher Review

A meeting between Fowler and Thatcher involving Peach in July 1986 had concentrated on efficiency. Competitive tendering for support services was to be pursued with more vigour. Resource allocation (RAWP) policies were to be reviewed in order to encourage patient referral to London hospitals, and changes were to be sought in consultants' contracts that 'ensured they perform the duties expected of them and the merit award system to be reformed so as to reward the efficient use of NHS resources as well as academic excellence.'[105]

In order to pursue the matter further, in September 1986 the Prime Minister invited the regional chairmen and one or two managers to dinner at Downing Street, where a number of chairmen made short but well-prepared presentations about progress in generating greater efficiency (income generation, supply, building programmes, staffing, etc.). Mrs Thatcher listened politely for a while until the mood suddenly changed. 'Why is it,' she asked, 'that with all the extra investment, waiting lists have gone up?' She made it plain that she was not impressed and wanted more action.[106]

By the end of 1986, Mrs Thatcher was asking more radical questions about the long-term future of the NHS. If neither a patient nor their GP was in a position to make an informed choice, there was little pressure to improve standards in healthcare, she asserted. If funding does not go to the hospital that the patient has chosen, the better hospitals will not have the resources to treat the patient.

By January 1987, Stowe and his policy team had prepared a highly confidential paper to send to Number 10, entitled *Towards a Better Healthcare: a Case for Change*.[2,57,71] It explored a comprehensive range of options for the future, and was regarded by Stowe as being highly contentious. These options included a tax-based system aimed at reducing or preventing an increase in the tax burden, and private health insurance (and tax incentives to encourage take-up) which might also take the pressure off the exchequer and reduce Government involvement in the provision of services. Patient charges were discussed (hotel costs, access to GPs and consultants, vaccinations, etc.), as was the potential for private capital investment. The paper also explored the arguments that might support the creation of an independent corporation, which not only could be given a great deal of discretion to provide services in terms of its day-to-day operation, but could also be contracted to deliver a specific package of services in a cost-effective way. The paper saw a very real advantage in distancing the operation and management of the NHS from central government, but acknowledged that this would only work if the NHS had its own source of funding.

A report by American professor Alain Enthoven[52] recommending the creation of a health market was reviewed in the paper, and the sceptical conclusions of the Management Board discussions some 18 months earlier were reported.

An exchange of minutes between officials in December 1987 seems to capture the concerns about market ideas:

> I have tried to be positive. If the management and political will can be found, I do not think existing legal and accounting restraints need prevent us from introducing market elements into the process of planning and providing services. A full-scale internal market approach on the Enthoven lines could only be achieved if really fundamental

changes were pushed through. I am still doubtful whether an Enthoven-type model would give sufficient voice to the consumer, the patient.[71]

There was another meeting with Mrs Thatcher at the end of January 1987, which reached the following conclusions.

1 Money needed to go with the patient in order to make service providers more responsive to patient needs.
2 There should be more connection between demand for care, its cost and the method of paying for it.
3 One possibility was to link funding to the health stamp. However, people might see this as health tax in disguise.
4 Health authorities might be given incentives to raise money from their local community or firms might buy extra services for employees.
5 Some form of Independent National Health Corporation should be considered.
6 Public opinion needed to be softened up before the next Parliament, when any reforms that the Government decided upon would be implemented.[71]

Fowler went away to ponder this discussion. Peach was not involved. This was high policy. However, Fowler was quite attracted to the idea of an Independent Corporation to manage the NHS on a day-to-day basis, although Mrs Thatcher was opposed to the idea. It was not that she did not think such a step could improve the management of the NHS, but rather that she worried about what people would say. What would be next? Privatisation?[29]

In her memoirs, Margaret Thatcher recalls these discussions as being 'very theoretical debates'.[34] She did not think 'we were yet in a position to advance significant proposals for the manifesto or even at an early stage in the next Parliament.' The political climate was not right for radical change. 'We can't do it,' she told Kenneth Stowe.[107] However, she was briefly tempted by the idea of another Royal Commission.

Although the Government was not in the mood for radical changes to the NHS, Kenneth Clarke was beginning to express an interest in pulling out of national pay bargaining, which for some represented a really big step.[107] What none of them had anticipated was the major financial crisis which would come to a head immediately after the election and force the Thatcher NHS Policy Review.

Fowler retires: John Moore takes over

In June 1987 the Conservatives won the General Election and Norman Fowler retired. He had been Secretary of State for six years. Ken Stowe recalls:

> Norman Fowler and I had a very, very good relationship in which we absolutely trusted each other. He knew that I would be thinking about how to do this, and I knew that he would want me to be thinking about how to do this and, therefore, I had no inhibitions about carrying my thinking as far as I could and then going back to him and saying, 'this might be a way to do it'.[2]

Peach said:

> Normal Fowler was a veteran by the time I arrived, but I was drawn
> into Norman Fowler's meetings because he had a sort of crisis meeting
> on a regular basis and that meant I was there to listen and answer.
> They were short term, they were mainly concerned with what was
> happening next week or the next two weeks, or what are we going to
> announce and so on. They were communications orientated.[82]

Hart contrasts Fowler with Clarke:

> Norman Fowler committed lots of effort to the political and presenta-
> tional side of the NHS. Of course Kenneth Clarke did, too, but he was
> also deeply interested in how management should be reformed and
> had very clear ideas about that.[39]

Fowler's successor was John Moore, who walked straight into a financial
crisis. Tony Newton stayed on as Minister of Health and as Chairman of the
Management Board.

John Moore, Secretary of State, 1987–88

John Moore came from a working-class background, was a London School
of Economics graduate and was a member of the Kennedy clan while
working in the USA as a financial analyst. He was elected MP for Croydon
Central in 1974, and he stood down in 1992. Between 1979 and 1987 he
held posts in Energy, the Treasury and Transport. He was appointed
Secretary of State for Social Services in June 1987 and was pitched straight
into the Thatcher Review and a major financial crisis. He was taken ill in
November 1987 and never really recovered. His job was split in 1988 and he
took over Social Security. He was created Lord Moore of Lower March in
1992.

Financial problems

Throughout Peach's term in office the NHS had been under substantial financial
strain. Cost improvement programmes were used to shore up deficiencies in the
national funding for wage awards. Health authorities extended the payment
period for creditors as a means of managing their cash flow. Beds began to close in
significant numbers. Financial growth was low in many health districts and non-
existent in others.

The proportion of the country's gross domestic product spent on health had
declined in England from 5.5% in 1981–82 to 5.1% by 1986–87, and was to stay
below 6% until 1992, only to fall back again for the rest of that decade.[108]

The cash problems that the south-east in particular was suffering were due in
part to the impact of the redistribution of revenue under the resource allocations
(RAWP) formula. By the late 1980s this policy had significantly reduced the
revenue gap between the north and the south of England. Eleven of the 14
regions were by then within 3% of either side of the target. Those out of line were

East Anglia, which was 3.99% away from target, and Northeast Thames, which was still 7.29% above target.

In the summer of 1987, regional chairmen and their general managers began to express serious concerns about the financial problems inside the NHS. If the books were to balance, either somebody would have to find more cash or services would have to be cut.

Plans were being drawn up to close wards and severely curtail non-emergency surgery. Priority services would inevitably be affected. John Moore and his ministers tried to calm the regions down. Although they acknowledged that there was pressure in the service, they argued that the financial settlement had been quite good in 1987–88 and much more could, they thought, be done to increase cash-releasing cost improvement programmes. Moore thought it 'bizarre to find the NHS success story masquerading as failure'. By this time the newspapers had picked up the theme and day after day there were headlines about cuts, closures and patients who had died. The regional general managers told the NHS Management Board that the service was approaching a spiral of despair.[109]

On 30 September 1987 a small group of regional chairmen and managers discussed the crisis with Tony Newton. Official regional reports showed a problem but not a crisis, and were thought to understate the problems. The following options for action were agreed upon:[110]

1 narrowing down central priorities for action
2 clearing roadblocks to efficiency in the acute sector, including consultant contracts
3 stopping some clinical services
4 limiting the expansion of doctors and nurses
5 introducing charges to patients and developing income generation
6 persuading doctors to help instead of shroud waving
7 reducing cost improvement programme targets.

Regional chairmen later made it very clear to John Moore that 'the difficulties previously reported are persisting and the overall position deteriorating, savings generated by Cost Improvement Programmes (CIP) were being largely consumed by non-planned demand'. Moore said that he would welcome an informed debate but that 'public appeals for more money would hinder rather than help negotiations with the Treasury.'[110]

One regional chairman in particular wondered whether the NHS Management Board should be removed as part of any financial rescue package. They seemed in his judgement to be making little impact on the service and were 'almost invisible except for the regular weekly letter from Mike Fairey about Information Technology!'. A division was beginning to be visible between the Civil Service and the other members of the board who wanted to take the Treasury on in a fight for more cash.[110]

Many hoped that John Moore would secure a better than expected settlement from the Treasury in the Public Expenditure Survey (PES) round, but his speech to the Conservative Party Conference in October gave them little hope. He promised no cash but a determined attempt to sweep away myths and sacred cows. He saw the future as depending on a closer partnership with the private sector, more independent contractors, income generation and other commercial ventures. It was later suggested that Moore had not fought all that hard for cash for the NHS, and had been congratulated in Cabinet by Nigel Lawson for being so reasonable in the negotiations.[111]

Christopher France, Permanent Secretary, 1988–91

Christopher France was born in the East End of London and attended the same school as Victor Paige, although four or five years later. His father was in the Navy, and although his mother was working she was determined that he would not be evacuated, so she and Christopher moved around the country with her jobs. He was later to spend part of the war in a Soldiers', Sailors' and Airmen's Families Association children's home in Hertfordshire. Christopher France began his working career as a schoolmaster, but decided that although he enjoyed teaching, he wanted a change. He had always been interested in the House of Commons, and on seeing an advertisement in the *Economist* for a House of Commons clerkship, he applied. On the application form there was a box to tick for the Home Civil Service. He was offered both jobs, but the First Civil Service Commissioner advised him to join the Civil Service. France had a philosophy, politics and economics degree from Oxford. At this time the Treasury was interested in people who were economically literate, and France was placed here, where he remained for 20 years.

In 1980 he was seconded to the electricity industry, and then spent three years in the Ministry of Defence. In 1984 he went to the DHSS to head the Policy Group. In 1986 he was appointed to the social security side of the DHSS as second Permanent Secretary, and a year later he took charge of the DHSS on the social security side as Permanent Secretary.

When the DHSS divided into Health and Social Security in 1988, France became Permanent Secretary for Health, and he remained in the Department of Health until 1992, when he went back to the Ministry of Defence for his last three years in the Civil Service.

Christopher France and his policy team tried hard to assist Moore in turning his ideas from the party conference about a different public/private mix into a working reality. He asked for policy work on the following:[71]

- proposals to reduce barriers between the private and public sectors and to increase the ability of health authorities to trade services even though the private sector would not welcome the competition
- outright privatisation of services was not to form part of the short-term agenda
- the need to follow up the point made by Len Peach about presenting the cost improvement programmes in a positive light
- health promotion to be an important part of a new strategy
- making cross-border flows easier (but the Enthoven model was not to be adopted)
- the extension of private health insurance, in order that the issue could be raised with the Chancellor.

In December, France, who would succeed Kenneth Stowe as Permanent Secretary in January 1988, tried to pin Moore down to define more closely the essence of the policy debate:

> Underlying all these points is the fundamental question: are we aiming to plan the provision of services or is it considered that a market mechanism will actually provide a more efficient service and one that is more responsive to customer demands? Did the introduction of a fully-fledged version of the internal market mean the end of a managed Hospital and Community Health Service?[71]

Like his predecessor, France did not favour primary legislation. 'My own preference,' he advised John Moore, 'was to avoid structural change unless it is essential to some clear purpose. There was a tendency in large organisations to change structures before the fruits of the last change had ripened.'[71]

Financial crisis, 1987–88

The outcome of the Public Expenditure Survey (PES) negotiations had been announced on 3 November 1987, but cut little ice with the NHS, which expected real growth to be well under 1%. The £707 million on offer was simply not enough and health ministers knew this. To make matters worse, there was a 'cock-up' in the deal with the Treasury as a result of a misunderstanding about the commitment to fund the previous year's Review Body awards. The civil servants who could not reach an agreement after a row referred the matter to ministers. John Moore discussed the problem with the Chancellor, who gave no ground at all. John Moore elected not to fight. There was deep embarrassment all round. Four options for coping were discussed at a highly confidential meeting on 13 November 1987:

- cutting clinical services
- no wage awards the next year
- bigger cost improvement programmes
- stopping the capital programme.

In November 1987, Tony Newton and his ministerial colleagues met in Cambridge with regional chairmen and some of the leading general managers (John Moore was ill). John James, the civil servant who had led on the PESC negotiations (and later migrated into NHS management), reported that the outcome for the following year was real-term growth of 1.8% (if one believed that the allowance for NHS inflation and pay awards was adequate, which few did, including ministers). Of the balance, much was already earmarked for AIDS, a wholly unforeseen new demand on the NHS, and acute-sector pressures, including waiting lists. The GDP level of investment was programmed to decrease from 5.2% to 5.1%.[110]

Ian Mills, the Director of Finance, reported on his review of the state of health authorities' finances. It was a bleak, if patchy, picture. A likely recurrent overspend of £12 million could be covered on a non-recurrent basis to balance the books, but most of the deficit would carry forward into the 1988–89 expenditure base. In about 25% of all health districts, services would have to be reduced in order to keep within cash limits, and in another 25% service rationalisation was needed to protect service capacity within the funding available. 'The NHS has,' Mills reported, 'been living beyond its means for some years and was technically insolvent at the end of 1986–87.'[110, 112]

Sir Donald Wilson, the Mersey Chairman, talked about the potential consequences of a further financial squeeze in the high-profile districts. Sir James Ackers, Chairman of the West Midlands Region, supported him and explained that a natural retrenchment of 2% meant a loss of 15 000 jobs. This would, he claimed, stretch the loyalty of DHA members and Tory MPs too far, particularly as it would have to be implemented against the solid and organised opposition of the hospital consultants.[114]

Newton and his colleagues (including Edwina Currie who, as a former health authority chairman, had a good feel for the issues involved) acknowledged the problems and accepted that some developments would have to be slowed down. However, they wanted greater efficiency and no reductions in service levels. They did not want publicly visible changes that could be labelled as cuts. They acknowledged that the lengthy consultation process that had to be undergone prior to service change needed review, and they promised to see if anything could be done that would speed up the process. Newton was very reluctant to agree to any more DHA mergers – an issue that he said needed to be handled with extreme care – even though they offered substantial savings. He insisted that any ideas for mergers must be discussed with him before being explored locally.[110] He was even more resistant to limiting the range of services provided by the NHS, and would only agree to informal discussions between regional officers and his officials on the matter. He urged more cost improvements and pinned a lot of hope on the impending issue of a circular on income generation in the NHS. He understood that it was unlikely that pay and price inflation could be held within 4.5% without 'unacceptable consequences.' The application of the resource redistribution policy (RAWP) formulae within regions was to be pursued with discretion. 'The situation,' he explained, 'reflects both the almost unlimited demand for healthcare, and the need for the Government to control public expenditure, in the interests of maintaining a strong economy and thus creating the wealth on which future spending will depend.'[115]

Each region was asked to produce an immediate handling plan for discussion with ministers. They did not want the national assessment to be disclosed on the grounds that it might impact on pay negotiations. Ministers viewed the issue as a problem to be handled rather than as a crisis, and this proved to be a major misjudgement on their part. The regions left the meeting feeling very dissatisfied, and later that day they agreed to find every opportunity to re-emphasise their message. Chairmen were later to ask for an away-day with ministers to explore the problems in more depth and gain a better understanding of their ideas about the future. They were particularly anxious about the public handling of what was a very gloomy scenario. They would not support any ideas for a national celebration on the fortieth anniversary of the NHS.

The public protests continued. Newton pressed the Treasury for more cash. He seemed to be making progress in the run-up to Christmas, but was getting little support from Number 10, particularly in the light of the intervention by the Presidents of the Royal Colleges. The Presidents of the Royal Colleges had been getting more and more anxious about the funding crisis throughout the autumn of 1987, and began to write to the press and demand meetings with ministers. In December 1987 they issued a press release:

> Every day we learn of new problems in the NHS – beds are shut, operating theatres are not available, emergency wards are closed, and essential services are shut down in order to make financial savings. In spite of the efforts of doctors, nurses and other hospital staff, patient care is deteriorating. Acute hospital services have almost reached breaking point. Morale is depressingly low. An immediate overall review of acute hospital services is mandatory. Additional and alternative funding must be found. We call on the Government to do something now to save our Health Service, once the envy of the world.'[116]

This statement, which some in the Department of Health would have encouraged, might well have been instrumental in helping Newton in his negotiation with the Treasury and Downing Street.

He eventually succeeded just before Christmas 1987 in securing an additional £100 million, which included £13.3 million for the damage caused to many NHS buildings by the great storm which hit the south of England on 15 and 16 October. The price was a significant sharpening up of the oversight of health authority finances and activity levels. The deal had been effectively struck between Newton and John Major at the Treasury.

Len Peach had allowed Ian Mills, the Director of Finance, to lead the discussions with ministers and the NHS throughout this period, which was very much his style. However, Peach did get drawn into one particularly poignant case of a small baby named James Barber, barely a few weeks old, who was waiting for 'hole in the heart' surgery at Birmingham Children's Hospital. The operation had been cancelled five times in six weeks due to staff shortages. The parents took the hospital to court and petitions and demonstrations began to be organised. Peach was in Stafford presenting prizes to nurses when he was caught up in a demonstration by the mothers of patients on waiting lists at the Birmingham Children's Hospital. He persuaded them that he was trying to solve the problems.[82]

Mrs Thatcher is said to have been particularly incensed at the events in Birmingham. She, and others at the time, thought that they had been set up by local doctors who had resisted the transfer of some of their patients to other units with spare capacity. The consultants claimed to have been told by their local chairman to stop speaking out about the plight of patients. The media had a field day, as they did with the closure of intensive-care beds in Manchester and when nurses from St Thomas's Hospital picketed the Houses of Parliament.

The Presidents got their meeting with the Secretary of State in January 1988. They came away optimistic, but their hopes were quickly knocked on the head by an emphatic denial from the Treasury that there would be any more money for the NHS. Despite these public denials, the Chancellor of the Exchequer had privately concluded that 'we had reached the point where the pressures to spend more money on the NHS were almost impossible to resist.'[117] He, too, was pushing for a fundamental review.[118]

In the mean time, John Moore was developing ideas of his own, including a health index that would measure over time the extent to which the health of the community was improving.

Health Services Supervisory Board: winding up

The Supervisory Board had met only intermittently during 1986 and 1987, and it no longer played a significant role inside the Department. In April 1987, Fowler had insisted that papers relating to the Public Expenditure Survey round should not be circulated without his express approval, and this ban included the Supervisory Board. Meetings planned for April, May and June 1987 were all cancelled. Sir Raymond Hoffenberg, who was by now at serious odds with the Government about funding (having likened health policy to applying elastoplasts to erupting sores until the whole body was covered in plaster), had asked the CMO, 'May I ask about the HSSB? There have been no meetings for four or five months and I still have blocked out the first Monday in each month – need I still do so?' The reply came, 'Don't hold the dates.'[119]

Soon after his appointment as Secretary of State, John Moore restyled the Board's role 'to provide a small forum for focusing on strategic direction and development of the Department's responsibilities across the board.'[119] It had now become explicitly advisory and far removed from its founding purposes, which included oversight of the NHS Management Board. The membership stayed the same, but meetings were to be held on a quarterly basis.

John Moore chaired the meeting in January 1988, which was held at the new headquarters in Richmond House immediately opposite 10 Downing Street. They discussed the work of the Board, the emerging 'Strategy for Health' and the spring planning guidelines. The Board never met again. Papers were prepared for meetings in March and June, but both were cancelled.

Kenneth Clarke took over from John Moore in July, and it was he who finally announced the winding up of the Board in January 1989. As Roy Griffiths put it at the time, 'The Board has fulfilled a major task in overseeing the establishment of the Management Board and the introduction of general management. It provided ministers with a valuable forum in which to discuss broad strategic issues.'[119]

The trouble was that ministers had their own style of working and behaved very differently. As Chris France explains, 'The reason the HSSB faded away was that John Moore did not want to be advised in that particular form.'[120]

Len Peach was more robust and probably nearest the truth: 'The Supervisory Board was really a waste of time. Essentially what happened to it was that ministers got bored with it. They had already heard the debates beforehand.'[82]

The Thatcher NHS Review, 1988

The pressure on Mrs Thatcher and her ministers to do something about the NHS had been growing as the public and professional criticisms increased. She had discussed a major review with John Moore in July 1987, but at that stage wanted him to concentrate on trying to ensure better value for money from the existing system. Putting even more extra money in might ease the pressure, but Thatcher in particular had come to regard the NHS as a bottomless financial pit:

> Many district health authorities which ran hospitals overspent in the first half of the year and then cut back by closing wards and postponing operations. They promptly blamed us, publicising the sad cases of

patients whose operations had been postponed, or, in the ghoulish phase used amongst doctors, shroud waving.[34]

In attacking the Government in the way they did, the medical profession had upped the political ante to the point where Mrs Thatcher had to respond. As Chris France put it, 'If there was a group of people responsible for triggering Mrs Thatcher's reforms it was they, because they raised the temperature to the point where she had to find a safety valve to let the steam out.'[120]

Mrs Thatcher announced the decision to have a review on *Panorama*, the BBC's leading current affairs television programme, on 25 January 1988. Chris France, the Permanent Secretary, was watching the programme at home that evening. 'Now that is interesting, 'he said to his wife, 'I shall no doubt hear about it in due course.'[120] Although they had had no warning of the announcement, it was not all that much of a surprise. France had consulted Moore in December 1987 about the idea of the Prime Minister chairing a small group of ministers in a policy review of the NHS. Moore told his officials that he was strongly opposed to such an idea.[71]

The review was conducted largely behind closed doors by a group of five ministers, namely Margaret Thatcher, Nigel Lawson and John Major from the Treasury, and John Moore and Tony Newton from the DHSS, who were replaced halfway through by Kenneth Clarke and David Mellor. Junior ministers were not directly involved and, according to Edwina Currie, had 'to hassle to get access to papers.'[101] Regional chairmen were not pleased about their exclusion either. The best they achieved was a submission of evidence and a day with John Moore on 16 March to explore the issues.[110] It was not a formal committee of the Cabinet. They planned to have something ready for the party conference in October of the same year. Roy Griffiths was a regular attender, and there were a number of meetings at Chequers for selected advisers and others drawn from the NHS. They had plenty of papers to get at. The paper prepared by Stowe in 1987 had covered the essential options.[71] David Willetts at the Centre for Policy Studies had been working hard for some months at the behest of Mrs Thatcher and had plenty of ideas for change. In addition to this, 12 back-up papers were commissioned. Accordingly to John Major,[121] Lawson and Moore were both keen to be brave and to do something to solve the problem, and after initial reluctance Margaret Thatcher agreed.

She had set herself four principles at the outset of the review:

> There would be a high standard of medical care available to all regardless of income, users should have the greatest possible choice, any changes must result in genuine improvement in healthcare, not just higher incomes for those working in the service, and finally decision making must be devolved to a point as close to the patient as possible.[34]

The early discussions seemed to have focused on three particular ideas:

1 the setting up of American-style health maintenance organisations led by GPs, to be called local health funds
2 the introduction of a special health tax with scope for individuals to opt out and pay a lower rate of tax

3 extensive management reforms of the existing system to provide a bigger role for the private sector.

Everyone seemed to agree that money should follow the patient and that competition would improve both quality and efficiency.[122]

John Moore pushed the private health insurance argument hard, and the early discussions at least appeared to have the ear of Mrs Thatcher. Nigel Lawson, the Chancellor of the Exchequer, showed some early interest but eventually came out firmly opposed to the idea. It was very much against the underlying philosophy of neutrality in taxation, and it would be very expensive to give relief to the 5.5 million people who already had health insurance. There was also a danger that once the principle had been conceded in health, the pressure would grow for relief in other areas, such as education.[123]

The Treasury had also concluded that the funding systems based on private health insurance in use in other countries offered few if any advantages, and would simply involve jumping out of the frying pan into the fire. The NHS was a very good means of controlling public expenditure in this field. Lawson was quite keen to increase NHS charges, but Mrs Thatcher thought that this would be too unpopular with the electorate.

However, the ideas about internal markets, which had been trailed by Alain Enthoven[52] some three years earlier, and which might drive efficiency, were considered worthy of more discussion and possible experimentation. They were encouraged to pursue this line by a paper written by Ian Mills, the Director of Finance.[124] In it he argued that the resource management programme in the NHS would, if the experiments were successful, facilitate the privatisation of large parts of the NHS hospital activity, or even complete hospitals. Health authorities could become purchasers of services rather than providers. It would open the door to a voucher system for use in the public or private sectors, under which the Government might provide a sum which individuals could top up. It would also ease the introduction of an insurance-based system.

Although the review was carried out in private, the arguments leaked into the public domain in the spring of 1988. Opinion was of course divided about the value of private health insurance and competition. The health professions reacted strongly. The Royal College of Nursing, which had just had a major wage award, expressed itself as 'radically opposed to any schemes that are perceived to threaten the NHS.'[38] The nurses wanted the Government to spend more on the NHS. Others demanded that the review should concentrate not on cost, but instead on medical effectiveness, and quoted a research paper published in the *New England Journal of Medicine*, which suggested that competition in health services increased mortality: 'In a fierce competitive environment, corners are cut and the quality of clinical care suffers.'[126]

In July 1988, with the NHS Review stuck in interminable arguments, Mrs Thatcher took the decision to split the DHSS into two. It was just too unwieldy, and John Moore was not coping.[34] John Moore took over Social Security and Kenneth Clarke came in as Secretary of State for Health. Clarke was not one of Mrs Thatcher's confidants, but had the benefit of knowing the NHS from his earlier stint as Fowler's number two.

> Margaret and John had briefed me with enthusiasm about how
> exciting it was going to be, and John in particular said that he had

got Margaret to promise him that tax relief for private health insurance was going to be the policy, and he and Margaret did not think the tax payer should pay for anybody who could afford to pay for themselves. The secret was to give tax relief for health insurance and then everything would sort itself out.[38]

Clarke took a different view and sided with Nigel Lawson and the Treasury. Eventually he and Lawson would concede a little ground by allowing tax relief on health insurance, but only for the elderly. In an interview, Clarke said 'I remember walking down the corridor with Nigel saying we have got as far as we are ever going to get, we should go quietly and get on with the health reforms.'[38]

As 1988 progressed, the review became so bogged down that Mrs Thatcher suggested that John Major should take over the Chair in order to make progress. He wisely demurred.

At this point it appears that Clarke took over the responsibility for bringing the review to a conclusion. The review team rarely met in full, but the Prime Minister maintained a keen ongoing interest. She understood the politics of getting it right, and had given up on ideas to reform funding mechanisms.[34]

Shortly after taking up office, Clarke had disappeared on holiday to Galicia in Spain. He was bird watching and reading the stack of papers he had taken with him about the NHS Review. He had chosen a difficult time to be away.

Reporters and nurses were wandering around airports all over Spain with wanted posters and rewards for finding the missing minister. As Clarke read his brief he warmed to the idea of fundholding. It was in his view the key to the purchaser side of the internal market. GPs would be better than managers at sorting out patients' needs and getting the priorities right. He came back to the UK with his ideas sketched out on a scruffy piece of paper.[38] Most managers and some of his ministers were deeply sceptical about them.

The idea that hospitals should be contracted out either individually, or in groups, through charities, privatisation or management buyouts appeared quite early in the review, as what were named 'self-governing hospitals'. The idea was regarded as extremely radical and a challenge to deeply engrained models of public sector management.[34] NHS trusts, as they eventually emerged, appear to have their roots in the independence of the teaching hospitals in the early days of the NHS, when their Boards of Governors had been accountable directly to the Department of Health rather than to the Regions. Ian McColl, a surgeon at Guy's Hospital (and later Parliamentary Private Secretary to John Major), had discussed this idea with David Willetts, now an MP, but then policy adviser to Mrs Thatcher.[111] However, according to Clarke, it was he and Mellor who worked the basic idea into a working proposition, and Clarke claims for himself the decision to call the hospitals 'trusts'. It sounded in his view more caring and friendly than 'self-governing hospitals', although the institutions of course had no element of trust status about them at all in the strict legal sense.[125] It was Clarke's private secretary Andy McKeon who suggested putting NHS in front of the trust title as a means of reinforcing their place within the NHS. Thus hospitals opted out of health authority control but remained within the NHS.

Another idea that rumbled around during the review, according to Mrs Thatcher,[34] but which never really emerged as policy, was the idea of rewarding performance with cash.[126] NHS growth could be top-sliced by the Department and allocated to those who met Government targets. This was another Thatcherite idea that would have to wait for Blair's Labour Government before it was implemented.

Inside the Department of Health, Clarke had pulled together a small team of 'really dedicated enthusiasts, led by Andy McKeon, his private secretary. Duncan Nichol was thick as thieves with us'. Clarke describes this team as 'young, not set in their ways, ambitious, bright, but bored with what they were doing.'[38] This was not the heavyweight team from the policy division, although they undoubtedly knew what was going on and no doubt offered more than an occasional steer to their more junior colleagues.

Clarke remains sharp in his criticism of the Department of Health at this crucial stage:

> When it came to the reforms, the most important changes in the Health Service since 1948, there were no people available to work on it. They were all far too busy doing whatever they were doing at that moment. I kept going on at my Permanent Secretary about the fact that we employed 6000 officials and I had no idea how we employed the time of more than about 100 of them.[38]

Although it is almost certainly true that the Department of Health would have been collectively very wary about radical reform, the senior team did kick in as the White Paper was worked up in detail. Clarke himself led the drafting team, which included Jonathan Hill (his special adviser), Strachan Hepple and David Clarke from the Policy Division and Andy McKeon, his private secretary. As the details progressed, other teams were created, including NHS trusts (Karen Caines), GP fundholding (Geoffrey Podger) and legislation (John Thompson).

Two other people played a key role according to Clarke. The first was Sheila Masters, who had succeeded Ian Mills as the Director of Finance for the NHS and who was, according to him, 'as tough as old boots but who understood money and financial control.'[38]

The other key player was the Cabinet Office Deputy Secretary, Richard Wilson, who had to keep an accurate record of the 'increasingly belligerent, argumentative and wild meetings in Number Ten'[38] between Thatcher, Lawson, Clarke and sometimes Major, as they clarified their minds about the purchaser/provider split. 'Margaret Thatcher,' according to Clarke, 'was fairly resistant the whole time and kept wanting to go off to her pet businessmen and produce alternative theories of her own; she did not trust us to do all of this.'[38] A number of sources confirm that discussions were very robust in their final stages, and even Clarke sometimes came back to his office 'in need of a restorative drink after a hand-bagging by the Prime Minister.'[120] 'It was,' Clarke explained, 'the way Margaret Thatcher worked. Kenneth Baker had an even more torrid time with his education reforms.' Richard Wilson used to grade these discussions on the Richter scale so that Ken Clarke's team knew what to expect on his return to Richmond House.[38]

In the end the Clarke Review Team's own timetable of one year, which had been set by Mrs Thatcher, forced out a result. The Treasury eventually backed off in their opposition to fundholding, which they had maintained from the start. In Lawson's view, 'GPs should have nothing whatever to do with spending money.

Those who did spend money must be accountable finally to them.' The Government opted for organisational change within the existing funding structure. The only concession to the private sector was tax relief on private health insurance for pensioners.[127]

One argument, about the possible merger of health authorities and family health service authorities, continued right up to the printing of the White Paper before the Treasury withdrew its objections and agreed to continue the separation. A proposal to replace the close central government control of the NHS with a free-standing English Health Authority had been rejected in favour of an NHS Executive operating as a management body inside the Department of Health.[365]

Len Peach, as Chief Executive of the NHS, had played little direct part in the review of the NHS. He understood that the review was a matter of major strategy and policy, although he did at times 'wonder if he had been wasting his time with his current change agenda.'[82] He had pushed on with the by now well-established practical agenda of implementing the Griffiths Report. Changing the management culture and improving the management of human resources were his day-to-day priorities. In the summer of 1988 the restructuring of the nursing profession in England had started to go badly wrong. There were huge variations across the country in the application of the national grading agreement for nurses. The projected addition to the national pay bill was 15.5%. Peach had to insist that no nurse be told what their assessed grade was until the national position became clear and acceptable.[124] By October there were serious doubts that the issue could be settled in time for nurses to receive their back pay before Christmas.[128] Up and down the country this issue dominated management and trade union relationships, and was the source of much tension. It was settled after a fashion before Christmas, but the appeal processes went on for years. It was not until the summer of 1993 that the position was largely solved by offering buyouts to staff with appeals still pending.

While all this was happening, the new Permanent Secretary, Chris France, found himself going over old ground with the regional chairmen, who had again been seeking clarity about responsibilities and accountability.[120] At a meeting with ministers in March 1988 they had commented on 'an apparent confusion of responsibility within the Department'. France was commissioned to respond to Donald Wilson, then Chairman of the regional chairmen's group:

> The Department of Health is part of government, not part of the NHS. The nation's health would be a matter for government whether or not there was an NHS. Because the NHS is virtually entirely financed from voted monies, its management is a matter for government. There is an inevitable political dimension when it comes to the use to which resources provided by the taxpayer are put and the efficiency with which they are used. The importance to government of the NHS and its management is recognised by Len Peach's appointment as Second Permanent Secretary, who leads at the most senior level on management issues which affect the service. The political importance of the NHS is recognised by the Minister's place as Chairman of the Management Board.[129]

All this was to change in a matter of a few months.

In December 1988, the Secretary of State, Ken Clarke, lost one of his ministers, Edwina Currie, who was forced to resign in a fiasco over salmonella and eggs. Her outspokenness had made her an easy target.

The NHS Review concludes: *Working for Patients*

Although the review had moved away from fundamental changes to funding mechanisms, the planned changes to the NHS were very radical indeed. They introduced the internal market to the health sector, created a split between purchasers and providers, and introduced NHS trusts and GP fundholding. The money would follow the patient. All of this was to operate on 1 April 1991. No one knew exactly how it would work, and few thought it could be done in this timescale.

Health authorities of all kinds lost their local authority representation and were reorganised along business lines with executive and non-executive directors. At the centre, the Supervisory Board was replaced by a Policy Board, which first met on 7 July 1989.[119] The Management Board was remodelled as the NHS Executive, and would be chaired by the chief executive rather than a minister. The Family Practitioner Services came under the executive for the first time, and were made accountable to the regional health authorities.[131]

When Clarke presented his final version of the White Paper to Cabinet he made it plain that it would not be popular. There was going to be a major political row and the Government would have to fight to get their reforms in place.[111]

The plans for change were launched to the NHS and the public in a spectacular manner on 31 January 1989. Clarke sailed down from Westminster to the Limehouse studios in London's Docklands for a national teleconference. At the same event the NHS was introduced to its new Chief Executive, Duncan Nichol (paid as a Second Permanent Secretary on a three-year contract), while Peach watched quietly from the sidelines.

Peach had decided a short while before the launch that it was time for him to return to IBM. Introducing these changes needed a new set of skills, and in any case he was on the verge of missing out on stock options at IBM that were part of his retirement planning. He was liked and respected by the Civil Service, who admired his consensual approach. He relied heavily on good interpersonal relationships and could make an untidy context work.[2] He appeared more distant to the NHS and never really lost his image as the Personnel Director (which was, of course, deliberate on his part). He enjoyed his term of office.[82]

In December 1995, some years later, he was selected to be the Commissioner for Public Appointments, a sure sign of trust by the establishment.

The reform plans had a mixed reception. The professions were mainly negative, but the Institute of Health Services Management gave the plans the 'amber light'. They liked many of the ideas, but would have preferred a proper review of the resources of the NHS rather than yet another reorganisation.[132] The National Association of Health Authorities was very cautious, and wanted to be assured that the proposals were consistent with the maintenance of a comprehensive, publicly funded NHS.[133]

Despite the promise of more consultant posts, the BMA said very little publicly on the day, other than that they would consult their members. Clarke anticipated that this would mean opposition and said as much in his own media interviews. He attacked from the beginning.

Dr David Owen thought the proposals' more sensible provisions were smothered by others that would poison rather than reform the NHS. He was in favour of an internal market that would increase efficiency, but not an open market that would reduce standards. The plans represented, he claimed, an American solution without their levels of funding.[133, 134] Timmins, in *The Independent*, reports that 'Mr Willetts, the closest of the outsiders to the NHS Review, had asked a senior civil servant what he would do to the NHS if he was the Minister.' The reply was 'I'd either leave it entirely alone, because it is so politically dangerous, or I'd destabilise it and see what happened.'[130] Cynics thought that this was entirely possible.

Chapter 4

Timeline

1989

January

- The internal market proposals were announced. *Working for Patients*[94] was launched at videoconferences in eight English cities.
- The NHS Management Board was reorganised into the NHS Policy Board and NHS Management Executive.
- Duncan Nichol was appointed as Chief Executive of the NHS.

March

- Kenneth Clarke attended the Royal College of General Practitioners dinner and 'insulted' members.

June

- A total of 178 expressions of interest in trust status were lodged at the Department of Health.

August

- The BMA launched a poster campaign against the reforms.
- Iraq invaded Kuwait.

September

- The ambulance pay dispute started.

November

- The Berlin Wall was torn down.
- *Caring for People: community care in the next decade and beyond*[135] was published.

1990

March

- The ambulance pay dispute was settled.

April

- The BMA reluctantly agreed to a managerial presence on consultant selection and merit award committees as well as job plans for consultants. Doctors involved in management were to receive extra pay.

May

- Margaret Thatcher called in Ken Clarke and Duncan Nichol for a review of progress, in preparation for the introduction of the internal market into the NHS.

July

- The implementation plan for *Caring for People* was announced.
- Regional health authorities were reconstituted with executive and non-executive members.

August

- The BMA launched a poster campaign against the NHS reforms.

September

- District and special health authorities were reconstituted into new executive forms.
- Family health services authorities were reconstituted and made accountable to regional health authorities.

November

- Kenneth Clarke decided to move the NHS Executive to a new headquarters in Leeds.
- Margaret Thatcher resigned and John Major became Prime Minister.
- Kenneth Clarke moved to Education. William Waldegrave was appointed as Secretary of State with Virginia Bottomley as Minister for Health.
- Nelson Mandela was released from prison.
- Peter Griffiths, Regional General Manager of SE Thames Regional Health Authority, was appointed as Deputy Chief Executive

1991

April

- The internal NHS market was launched with 57 first-wave trusts and 306 GP fundholders.

June

- The report *Junior Doctors: the new deal*[136] was published.
- Kenneth Calman, Chief Medical Officer for Scotland, was appointed as Chief Medical Officer to succeed Sir Donald Acheson.

July

- New regional health authorities came into being.

September

- New district health authorities were created.
- Non-executive members of health authorities were paid for the first time.
- Sheila Masters, Director of Finance, produced a league table of regional performance.

October

- *The Patient's Charter*[137] was launched and reaffirmed that 'the Government believes there must be no change to the fundamental principles on which it (the NHS) was founded.'
- Peter Griffiths moved from the Department of Health to take over at Guy's and Lewisham NHS Trust.
- Andrew Foster (RGM Yorkshire) took up post as Deputy Chief Executive.

1992

January

- The NHS Executive announced the creation of its own Outposts to monitor the performance of NHS trusts, rather than regional health authorities.
- Sir Christopher France moved on to the Ministry of Defence. Graham Hart returned from Scotland to take over as Permanent Secretary at the Department of Health.

April

- Second-wave trusts and fundholding schemes were launched.
- The Conservatives won the General Election. Virginia Bottomley took over as Secretary of State, with Brian Mawhinney as Minister of Health. John Smith took over from Neil Kinnock as leader of the Labour Party. Kenneth Clarke became Home Secretary.

July

- The White Paper *Health of the Nation*,[138] issued by Bottomley, targeted five key areas for health improvement, namely coronary heart disease, cancers, HIV/AIDS and sexual health, mental health and accidents.

- Duncan Nichol was interviewed for the *Daily Mail* and created a political storm.
- The NHS Executive moved to Leeds.

September

- Andrew Foster left as Deputy Chief Executive to become Comptroller General at the Audit Commission.

October

- The Tomlinson Report[139] on the future of London hospitals was published.
- Alan Langlands was appointed as Deputy Chief Executive.

1993

February

- The London Implementation Group was set up.

March

- Regional health authorities were told to reduce their number of staff to 200 each. At their peak some had had over 1000 staff.

April

- The third wave brought the total number of trusts to 289.

May

- A series of speeches by Mawhinney and Nichol gave focus and strength to purchasing authorities in the NHS.

June

- UNISON was created out of a merger of the COHSE, NUPE and NALGO trade unions.

July

- The Maastricht Treaty was signed, leading to clash in the EEC.
- The Public Accounts Committee published highly critical reports on the management of the West Midlands and Wessex RHAs.

October

- Virginia Bottomley published the Jenkins Review[140] of the internal work and structure of the Department of Health.

November

- Trade unions mounted a protest march in London about the impact of the internal market on the NHS.
- The first unified budget and autumn statement were presented. A public-sector pay freeze was announced except for deals linked to productivity.

December

- Another restructuring was announced. The number of regional health authorities was reduced from 14 to eight on April 1994, and they were abolished altogether in 1996. A new NHS Executive was to be created including the eight regional directors.
- New NHS Policy Board was constituted.
- It was announced that district health authorities and family health services authorities could merge.

1994

January

- The Clothier Report (Allitt Inquiry) into deaths and injuries on the children's ward at Grantham and Kesteven General Hospital was published.[141]

March

- Sir Duncan Nichol retired as Chief Executive and took up the position of Chairman of International Healthcare Management at the University of Manchester.
- Alan Langlands was appointed as Chief Executive of the NHS Executive.

April

- A total of 419 NHS trusts (almost the whole of the provider system) and 9000 GP fundholders represented over half of all eligible practices and served 36% of the population.

May

- The *Review of the Wider Department of Health*[142] was published by Mrs Terri Banks.

Duncan Nichol, 1989–94

The search for a successor to Len Peach as Chief Executive was handled in traditional public service style with an advertisement and interview. Much to his displeasure, Roy Griffiths was not asked to join the selection committee.

Sir Graham Hart, Permanent Secretary, 1992–97

Graham Hart obtained a BA and became an Honorary Fellow of Pembroke College, Oxford. During this time he did a vacation job in a local hospital as a hospital porter, and knew that when he graduated from Oxford he wanted a job 'doing public service'. He was interested in the health service as an institution, and applied for both a Civil Service job and a place on the hospital administration scheme. He was offered both, and chose the Civil Service, putting the Department of Health as his first choice.

From 1962 to 1984 he worked his way through the Civil Service ranks within the DHSS and the Department of Health.

In 1982 he was the Director of Operations and for a short time Deputy Chief Executive of the NHS Executive. Between 1990 and 1992 he was Secretary of the Scottish Home and Health Department based in Edinburgh. He came back to the Department of Health as Permanent Secretary from March 1992 to 1997.

Sir Graham Hart was Chairman of the King's Fund until 2004.

Graham Hart, who had been Peach's deputy, did not apply for the job as the role model seemed to demand a manager from either the private sector or the public services, rather than a civil servant. 'I thought it should be very much from the NHS.'[39] A recommendation that Duncan Nichol, the RGM from the Mersey Region, who had been a part-time member of the Board since September 1995, be appointed eventually went up the line to Sir Robin Butler and Mrs Thatcher. There followed a frantic weekend of telephone calls dealing with the Prime Minister's questions and challenges. Would Nichol be any good in front of the television cameras? How would he cope with a Public Accounts Committee? Why had Chris West from Portsmouth not applied?[39] Donald Wilson, who was Nichol's chairman in Mersey, was reassuring, and eventually the appointment was approved and announced.

Sir Duncan Nichol, Chief Executive of the NHS Management Executive, 1989–94

Duncan Nichol was born in Bradford in 1941. From Bradford Grammar School he went to St Andrew's University in Scotland, where he read modern languages. He entered the NHS in 1963 as a graduate national trainee based at the King's Fund in London and the Northeast Thames

Region. His first substantive job was as Deputy Hospital Secretary at St Thomas's Hospital, and this was followed by a year in Chicago on a Sainsbury Scholarship. He returned to join the development and research team at St Thomas's, before moving to Manchester as Assistant Group Secretary to the United Manchester Hospitals with Andrew Scott. There followed a spell as House Governor at the Manchester Royal Hospital and, as teaching hospitals were designated around the City, he became first the deputy Group Secretary and then District Administrator in South Manchester. He became Area Administrator in Salford in 1987. He was appointed as Regional Administrator, and later Regional General Manager, of the Mersey Regional Health Authority in 1981. He inherited what was regarded at the time as a bottom-of-the-league region with many issues and difficulties in Liverpool in particular. Sir Donald Wilson became Chairman of the Board at around the time Nichol was appointed. They made a strong team and transformed the region into one of the better managed ones.

In 1985, Nichol joined the NHS Management Executive as a part-time non-executive director. He was appointed as Chief Executive of the NHS Management Executive in 1989 at the age of 48 years.

He became a Professor of International Healthcare Management at the University of Manchester in 1995. Since his retirement from that post he has become actively involved with the Home Office in both the management of the Prison Service and judicial appointments. In 2004 he was appointed Chairman of the Parole Board.

Duncan Nichol's appointment was warmly welcomed within the NHS. At last an NHS manager's talents had been recognised.

Getting the salary agreed proved to be difficult, as the salary that was agreed verbally was greater than the starting point for a second permanent secretary who was a new entrant to the Civil Service. In the end a secondment from the NHS was negotiated. It was much easier this way.

Duncan Nichol took over the reins from Len Peach in January 1989, and with his appointment came another major restructuring within the Department of Health following the publication of *Working for Patients*.[143] A new NHS Management Executive (NHS ME) was created, and an NHS Policy Board, chaired by the Secretary of State, replaced the Supervisory Board.

The terms of reference for the NHS Policy Board were focused on the creation of policy objectives for the NHS, to determine strategy within which the Executive would operate, and to monitor the Executive's performance. It had no brief with regard to the wider functions of the Department. The Chief Nursing Officer was excluded from the early meetings, which did not go down at all well with the nursing profession. Eventually the Director of Nursing was added to the team. The doubt about the need for a nurse at this level reflected similar questions at regional and district levels. Trevor Clay, the Secretary of the Royal College of Nursing, was so concerned that he launched his own public campaign, entitled 'Why is the NHS being run by people who do not know their coccyx from their humerus?'[109] In the event most senior teams had a senior nurse member, but the role was almost always supplemented with additional responsibilities, such as quality assurance.

NHS Management Executive, May 1989

Chief Executive	Duncan Nichol
Deputy Chief Executive	Graham Hart
Medical Director	Dr Ron Oliver
Director of Information Systems	Mike Fairey
Director of Nursing	Patsy Wright-Warren
Director of Finance	Sheila Masters
Director of Family Practitioner Services	Bryan Rayner
Director of Personnel	Peter Wormald
Director of Estate	Idris Pearce

NHS Policy Board, July 1989

Secretary of State (Chairman)	Kenneth Clarke
Deputy Chairman	Sir Roy Griffiths
Minister for Health	David Mellor
Parliamentary Under-Secretary for Health (Commons)	Roger Freeman
Parliamentary Under-Secretary for Health (Lords)	Lady Hooper
Chief Medical Officer	Sir Donald Acheson
Chairman, West Midlands RHA	Sir James Ackers
Professor of Paediatric Nephrology, Guys Hospital, London	Prof. Cyril Chantler
Chairman, South West Thames RHA	Julia Cumberlege
Permanent Secretary	Sir Christopher France
Chairman, Rover Group and Cadbury-Schweppes	Sir Graham Day
Chairman, Kingfisher Holdings, Deputy Chairman, British Aerospace	Sir Kenneth Durham
Chairman, British Steel	Sir Robert Scholey
Chief Executive, NHS Management Executive	Duncan Nichol

The Policy Board met for the first time in July 1989 in the Cathedral Room at Richmond House in London. From the beginning the meetings were dominated by Kenneth Clarke. A civil servant described the first meeting in the following terms:

> The Secretary of State dominated the meeting, both by his manner –
> he smoked a large cigar in a no smoking area – and by the way in
> which he used the opportunity to expose his own views, opening up
> certain areas for discussion whilst keeping others tight. The decision to

postpone the implementation of the Community Care policies by two years had been referred to the Board, but they had no opportunity to discuss it. Outside members tended to make a greater contribution than departmental members.[144]

We note, not for the first time, the distinction between those inside the Civil Service and those outside it.

Bob Scholey set the tone at an early meeting with a comment that the only way to ensure waiting lists were reduced was to make the performance-related pay of regional general managers directly related to this yardstick. 'If a few had to be shot for their failure it would be an example of the Department's commitment.'[145]

The majority of Nichol's Board came from within the Civil Service, but this situation was to change within the year.

The terms of reference for the new Management Executive were published following the first meeting of the new Policy Board in July 1989 'so as to establish the limits of ministerial responsibility for operational matters and define the Executive's role clearly enough for it to be able to establish its own identity.'[145]

Role of the Management Executive[145]

- To take central responsibility on behalf of ministers for the operation and management of the NHS.
- To set objectives for NHS authorities in line with overall ministerial priorities and within the resources allocated to it, and monitor their performance.
- To provide leadership to NHS management.
- To advise ministers and the Policy Board on the operation and management of the NHS.
- To carry out certain services at a national level in support of NHS authorities.
- To present the achievements of the NHS within the service and to the general public.

Management functions

- Issue of strategic and operational guidance to NHS authorities.
- Approval of regional objectives.
- Setting performance targets for NHS authorities.
- Developing and implementing policies for the improved use of revenue and capital resources and setting targets for cost improvements and income generation.
- Developing pay and personnel policies for endorsement by ministers and the Policy Board.
- Developing and advising on resource allocation policies.
- Developing and implementing accountability arrangements for regional general managers.
- The Chief Executive was accountable to the Policy Board and hence to the Secretary of State.[146]

These terms of reference were vague and almost contradictory. On the one hand, the Management Executive took central responsibility for the operation of the NHS (within the ministers' policy framework), and on the other they advised ministers and the Policy Board on the operation and management of the NHS. This was a headquarters team, which meant that it had to follow Civil Service traditions and do everything through ministers. There was no formal devolution of powers, and ministers retained the final accountability for the management of the NHS. At the time it did not seem to matter. It was such a revolutionary change – who wanted to quibble about the detail?

Nichol was given a very clear brief on his role and priorities from the Prime Minister. She wanted a recognisable public figure to take a firm grip of the NHS and its managers. 'I've had enough,' she told him, 'of the obstruction of the Permanent Secretaries and to some extent the reluctance of the politicians to make space for this job.'[147] According to Nichol, she invited Clarke, France and himself to a meeting very shortly after he had taken up his post, looked them straight in the eye and said 'Don't even think about getting in the way this time, otherwise it will be me you have to answer to.' She told Ken Clarke 'I want you off the television on things you should not be fiddling around with, like explaining why nurses are graded D in Netherwallop. That's nothing whatsoever to do with you – it's the Chief Executive's job.'[147]

Nichol told NHS Managers in an official circular that 'separating the role of managers from ministers will be a prime consideration. The implementation of policy will be the responsibility of the ME.'[148]

Mrs Thatcher clearly saw the Chief Executive as being the man in charge of the NHS, rather than an adviser to the Secretary of State. In the event Clarke and Nichol worked well together. France and Nichol quickly sorted out their respective territory, but only after a tussle about the introduction of the internal market. France wanted to chair an overarching committee to supervise progress, but Nichol would have none of it. He and his Executive had been appointed to do this and he wanted to do it with the NHS.[147] France accepted instead a small steering group to co-ordinate policy, which included the deputy Chief Executive and, as a face-saver, the Chief Nursing Officer.

Within 12 months Nichol had radically reshaped his team and, following Graham Hart's move to Scotland, brought in Peter Griffiths as his deputy, a man with a strong NHS background.

Nichol's term of office was dominated by the creation of an internal market in the NHS. It was a huge and complex undertaking that had to be achieved over a short timescale against a background of fierce opposition by the professions and trade unions. The health professions had opposed the planned reforms from the start. In April 1989, at the RCN Conference in Blackpool, the nurses had accused Clarke of undermining the principles of the NHS.[149] A few days later he had been taken behind a curtain in the Accident and Emergency Department at Hope Hospital, Salford, to be challenged by staff about his ideas for change. 'I have no time for a political barney,' he told them as he continued his visit, but that was exactly what he was going to get on all of his visits in the coming months.[113]

Nichol's Management Executive, 1990

Post	Holder	Background
Chief Executive	Duncan Nichol	NHS
Deputy	Peter Griffiths	NHS
Personnel	Eric Caines	Civil servant
Nursing	Michael Clark	Nurse
Information Systems	Michael Fairey	NHS
Operations and Planning	Mike Malone-Lee	Civil servant
Finance	Sheila Masters	Industry
Research and Development	Michael Peckham	Doctor
Family Health Services	Bryan Rayner	Civil servant
Medical Director	Diana Walford	Doctor
Property Adviser	Ian Oddy	Industry

As far as managers were concerned, Nichol had made it plain in March 1989 at a conference at Lake Windermere that 'the direction of change was fixed and the need now was to concentrate on the how, not the whether.'[150] Even at this early stage the first hospitals begin to express an interest in trust status, including a bid from all the hospitals in Oxford who wanted to combine as one. This was not judged to be helpful, as competition was what was required, not cosy cartels.

In the same month the BMA opened up another opposition front with a leaflet sent to GPs for circulation to their patients explaining that the Government was threatening to force doctors to limit the cost of the medicines they could prescribe. During his first few months Nichol found himself at the centre of a growing political storm.

In Ken Clarke the Chief Executive had a confident, tough but sometimes abrasive boss. Although Clarke respected the role of the Chief Executive, there was never any doubt that he was personally in charge of driving the new policies forward. NHS funding was still a problem, but Sheila Masters, the new Director of Finance, set about eradicating the underlying deficits in the system and introducing capital charges on to the balance sheets of NHS trusts prior to the introduction of the internal market. During 1989–90 she had assessed that two-thirds of district health authorities had deficits. The Department eventually found £81 million to bail out those with the highest creditor levels. By this time bed closures had bitten hard, and the earlier estimate of 3000 closures was regarded inside the department as almost certainly an underestimate.[151] In the Thames Regions little or no non-emergency surgery was taking place. Waiting lists were climbing.

Some of the financial pressure began to ease as increased investment coincided with the launch of the internal market.

NHS expenditure (public and private) as a percentage of gross domestic product (GDP)[27]

Year	Proportion of GDP (%)
1970	4.5
1980	5.6
1990	6.0
1998	6.8
2002	7.7

Source: Office of Health Economics (1997).

Internal market: smooth take-off

Nichol and Clarke had decided quite early on to aim for a smooth take-off for the new market on 1 April 1991. Neither of them could afford to run the risk of the NHS spinning out of control. The message went out to curb the enthusiasts and take it steadily. Nichol had argued for a steady state in year one, but Clarke took a slightly different view. He wanted 'a smooth take-off with no surprises',[152] but he also wanted change from day one.

There was an enormous amount of work to do by way of preparation. The NHS had to be able to specify and price services in a manner that it had never seriously contemplated before. The information foundation for this was woefully weak. Contracts had to be devised from scratch and then negotiated. There were thousands of questions to be resolved about the details of fundholding and the nature of trust status. Discussion papers and draft guidance notes flooded the system. The Executive and the wider Department of Health policy teams moved into top gear. An internal market for a large public service had never been created before. It was an exciting and intellectually satisfying challenge. In the second half of 1989 a series of working papers emerged from groups involving the Department and the regions, that filled in the detail about the reforms covering contracting, fundholding (called practice budgets at this stage), capital charges, medical audit and consultants' contracts. Assets of over £1000 had to be counted and valued. It was a massive job.

The preparations for change were disrupted when in September 1989 ambulance crews voted by 4 to 1 in favour of industrial action after rejecting a 6.5% pay offer. Other public sector workers had been offered more, and the police had been given 9.5%. A ban on overtime and rest-day working escalated into a full-scale strike in some parts of the country and also in London. This was the issue that forged the relationship between Nichol and Clarke. They talked most mornings about progress. They were determined from the beginning not to increase the offer because of the impact that it would have on negotiations with other groups and the funds available for growth, which would cushion the introduction of the new market. Clarke agreed that Nichol would lead with the media while he made sure that Parliament and the Cabinet were kept properly informed. This was particularly important because of the use of armed forces to provide emergency cover. Matters did get very serious indeed in London, and

Nichol and his team were well aware that people's lives were at serious risk.[147] The stakes were sharply increased when ambulance officers and controllers became involved. For a Permanent Secretary like Nichol to assume such a public role, including an interview with Jimmy Young, a popular radio programme presenter, in such a potentially explosive set of circumstances was highly unusual. For the most part this was how the dispute was handled, although Clarke did occasionally intervene directly with the media. Nichol saw no confusion of roles. The day-to-day operational decisions were inextricably bound up with the politics. Nichol bore the brunt of the day-to-day management of the dispute, but at the end of the day Clarke was in charge. Strategy, tactics, publicity and negotiations were all subject to his approval.

A settlement was finally reached in March 1990 on the basis of a two-year deal. Both sides claimed a victory, but the Department of Health probably had the most justification.

This dispute, although it brought Clarke and Nichol together, may ironically have prevented an independent identity for the Executive from developing early on in its history. The Executive was always working firmly within Clarke's shadow.

While all of this was going on, the pressure to stop the introduction of the internal market continued. Clarke had predicted a bitter fight, and he got one. The BMA launched what one MP called 'a thoroughly salacious and disgraceful advertising campaign'. A BMA video attacking the reforms was shown at public meetings, and in August a major poster campaign was launched. One ran as follows: 'What do you call a man who ignores medical advice? Mr Clarke.' The focus of the public challenge was self-governing hospitals and GP fundholding which, it was argued, would produce a two-tier service. This was raw politics with a dangerous edge to it. Many elderly people believed, wrongly, that they would be removed from their GP's list if they needed expensive drugs. Others thought that the creation of trusts would mean some hospitals 'opting out of providing free NHS healthcare'. The majority of the public believed that the reforms were designed to save money rather than to improve services. A series of five tracking surveys conducted by MORI for the Trent Region between September 1989 and November 1990 showed that over 70% of their residents held the view that the main aim of the Government's reorganisation was to reduce spending rather than to improve care.[109]

There were also many health professionals who, although they did not parade their views in public, were deeply sceptical and concerned about the reforms. They had a strong philosophical commitment to the public service and disliked the concept of a market in healthcare. Views such as these were common in the medical academic world, as the preamble to the World Summit on Medical Education in 1993 would make plain: 'The trend of medicine towards becoming a business enterprise is a serious diversion from its traditional commitment to caring and healing.'[153]

In November 1989, Clarke and his Policy Board had an extended debate about communications strategies in the NHS. It was the first of many such discussions. Explaining radical change to consumers and staff was challenging for the best organisations, but was even more difficult when there was also a high level of political controversy. A team of external consultants had been out and about in the NHS measuring current communications performance. The results were not impressive. They had proposed a major initiative designed to upgrade and improve communications with the staff of the NHS. They wanted every unit general manager in England to talk to every member of staff about the reform programme. Sir Robert Scholey had strongly supported some action, and described the employee research surveys that British Steel used on a routine basis to establish what their staff were thinking and how effectively their own messages had got through.[154] Duncan Nichol was also in favour, as he thought that any improvement would help managers to understand the reforms better, and thus be able to explain them to their staff. Leaflets explaining the reform programme began to appear all over the NHS, and during 1990 the Department of Health posted the booklet *The Reforms and You* to every household in the UK, at a cost of £2.75 million.[162] For the most part, staff and the public remained suspicious – these were political messages.

At the same Policy Board meeting, Anne Poole, the CNO, had a hard time with her plans to reform nursing, which had been worked out with the professions some months earlier. Everyone agreed that nurses needed management development. Roy Griffiths wanted more flexibility for local role definition, rather than fixed national models. Ken Clarke queried the need for nursing posts to be identified at every management level, and was particularly sceptical about the need for research nurses at district level. The CNO was not at all pleased with the rebuff she had received, and this view was no doubt shared with the other leaders of the nursing profession.

Behind the scenes, the negotiations with the BMA about the role that doctors would play in the internal market and the nature of their contracts had continued. Clarke insisted that managers must be permitted to join the selection panels for new consultant appointments and be members of the committees that made decisions about merit awards for senior hospital doctors. Merit awards were supposed to recognise exceptional skills among hospital consultants. Decisions about who would receive them had been made for years by doctors meeting in secret. There were four levels of award, namely A+, A, B and C. The highest award could double a consultant's salary.

Each consultant was to have a job plan that laid out his or her principal duties and commitments. The BMA had never been challenged in this manner before, and was particularly concerned about the plans to devolve consultants' contracts from the regional level to local hospitals (this despite the fact that consultant contracts of employment had been held at hospital level by the teaching hospitals since 1948 without any problems). They also objected strongly to the freedom of the new trusts to negotiate local pay. What would prevent, they asked, 'the board of directors of a Self-Governing Hospital (SGH) directing on an annual basis the detailed type of medical work which may or may not be carried out by consultant medical staff?'[155] There was much fire and bluster with meetings involving both sides breaking up for long private sessions. The Departmental negotiating team (which for the first time included an NHS manager) knew that it had little room for manoeuvre, and so did the BMA team, led at this stage by Anthony Grabham. Either an agreement could be reached or the Government's proposals would be enforced. Clarke was not a man for easy compromise. In separate meetings, although involving many of the same players, agreements were reached about the introduction of medical audit, which after much discussion Clarke was persuaded to incorporate into a reformed and expanded system of postgraduate medical education. The doctors had much to gain from these negotiations. It was not all loss.

The BMA did try at one stage to persuade Clarke to test the internal market with a pilot scheme, but he would have none of it. 'If I do that,' Clarke said, 'you will sabotage it.'[38] The doctors' opposition to the reforms ignited and sustained the public's anxieties about them. The BMA focused their attack on Kenneth Clarke, thus allowing Nichol to keep a lower public profile and his lines open to the professions. He talked regularly to the Royal Colleges and listened closely to their concerns. However, his relationship with the Joint Consultants Committee was nothing like as productive. After one particularly bad-tempered set-piece event he vowed never to go to one again.[147] Once the dust had begun to settle, he sought to build a new concordat with the medical profession. He was prompted in part to do this by Rudolf Klein, a leading academic, who had argued that the Government, at least in the eyes of the doctors, had torn up the 1948 concordat. According to Nichol this meant that 'the doctors would do the rationing as long as the Government did not get involved in asking questions about how they practised their trade.'[147]

Nichol knew that the market would open up difficult questions about clinical priorities, such as 'Why are we not doing renal dialysis on 65-year-olds?' He wanted the doctors on side when these questions hit the public domain. He was searching for 'an adult way, a grown-up way of taking collective decisions about priorities.'[147] It helped that the earlier experiments in involving doctors in resource management had been successful. The first six pilot resource management sites had been expanded to 50 hospitals by March 1990, and in the process they introduced significantly enhanced patient-coding systems, which was valuable for medical audit and research.[156] This initiative at least had the support of the doctors who as a group had been closely involved in its evolution. The language was eventually to shift to clinical management systems so as to bring in the other health professions.

In a parallel development, Nichol and his Director of Research, Michael Peckham, begin to lay the foundations of the health technology assessment programmes and reinforced the moves to evidence-based medicine. Nichol also encouraged multi-disciplinary postgraduate education with programmes of 'medicine for non-medical managers' and 'management for doctors'.

Sir Michael Peckham

Michael Peckham was born in 1935. He qualified at the University College Hospital Medical School and worked at the Royal Marsden from 1971 to 1986. He became Professor of Radiotherapy and cancer specialist, and was Director of Research and Development, NHS Executive from 1991 to 1995.

Mixed up in the negotiations about the reform programme was the unresolved issue of contracts and pay for general practitioners. Resignation was threatened regularly. Kenneth Clarke had inflamed the process somewhat at a dinner of the Royal College of General Practitioners in March 1989. According to Dr John Marks, Chairman of the BMA council, he made the comment 'I do wish the more nervous of our GPs would stop feeling nervously for their wallets every time I mention the word reform.'[111,157] It was a perfectly apt comment, but in the climate of the times it caused much offence. Eventually Michael Wilson, the GPs' leader, and Clarke did a deal late one evening in May. Five weeks later the membership voted against the deal, leaving Clarke no choice but to impose the contract against the will of the BMA. This he did in August 1989, when he wrote to all GPs about 'A New Contract.' The new contract increased the money paid to GPs through capitation fees, made higher payments for the care of patients over 75 years, and provided new fees for running health promotion clinics, teaching medical students and undertaking minor surgery. There was a new two-tier payment for reaching vaccination and immunisation targets, and help for GPs in areas of deprivation.

Virginia Bottomley, Secretary of State, 1992–95

Virginia Bottomley was born in Dunoon, Scotland in 1948. She was educated at Putney High School, and took a degree in sociology at Essex University, followed by an MSc in social administration at the London School of Economics and Political Science. She came from a family with strong health connections. Her father had been Chairman of St Thomas's Hospital in London.

She has worked as a researcher, a psychiatric social worker, a magistrate and Chairman of a Juvenile Court. She became a Member of Parliament for the South-West Surrey Constituency in 1984.

She has been a member of the Medical Research Council, and is a Governor of the London School of Economics, and a Freeman of the City of London.

Her parliamentary career began as PPS to Geoffrey Howe, who was Secretary of State for Foreign and Commonwealth Affairs (1987–88), and she then became Junior Minister in the Department of the Environment (1988–89). She began in the Department of Health as Minister of State in 1989, and became Secretary of State for Health in 1992. She later became Secretary of State for National Heritage (1995–97).

Cash to support the preparations for the reforms was made available in 1989–90 (£85 million) and £305 million in 1990.[158] Virginia Bottomley signalled her confidence in the preparations when she told Ann Widdecombe in February 1990 that 'the NHS would be ready to implement the basic elements of the reforms.'[159] However, reports began to emerge towards the end of March 1990 that Nichol was under pressure from managers to persuade Clarke to restrict any full-scale launch to a small number of pilot districts. The professional bodies and trade unions joined the call for a brake to be placed on the pace of reforms.[160]

Mrs Thatcher had watched the preparations closely and was far from satisfied. She wanted to discuss the possibility of slowing things down until after the election. The scale of the opposition had worried her, and according to Clarke she had been much taken by some advice she had received from Charlie Haughey, the Irish premier, that 'you can never win an election by fighting the doctors.'[39]

In June 1990, Mrs Thatcher summoned Kenneth Clarke and Duncan Nichol to a progress meeting in Downing Street. Peter Griffiths, the deputy Chief Executive, and Sheila Masters, the Finance Director, accompanied them. It was to prove to be a challenging event. Aligned on Mrs Thatcher's side of the table were three trusted heavyweight advisers who had been looking independently at the preparations for change, namely Sir David Wolfson, Sir Robin Ibbs and Lord Rayner. They had not been reassured by what they had found, and told Mrs Thatcher that they doubted whether health authorities and hospitals had the information technology, accounting systems and expertise necessary to cope with the changes.[34] Duncan Nichol delivered his prepared progress report. Mrs Thatcher's response was cool. 'All you have done is repeat back to me the principles of the reforms. I was the architect of those principles,' she said, 'I know them very well indeed. You are here to give me confidence that you know how to implement them.' At this point, according to Nichol, she opened her handbag and produced many pieces of paper, saying 'These are supposed to be contracts, 4000 contracts in London – the whole thing's a nonsense.'[147] An exasperated and angry Clarke took over the presentation at this point. 'Those people over there [the Prime Minister's advisers] know nothing about this and we are going to do it anyway, so what's it about, what's the point of this farce?'[147] The reforms, he argued, would develop. There was no need for detailed costing and information flow data at the start. He argued that on the political front it was better for the reforms to be started before the election so that the public could see for themselves that the criticisms and scaremongering were false.

'On your head be it,' was the Prime Minister's response as she left the room to go to another meeting. Timmins' account of this meeting[111] is essentially the same, although he reports on press coverage in advance of the meeting with headlines such as 'NHS retreat', which Clarke thought had been leaked in order to force a delay in implementation. The team retired back across the road to Richmond House feeling that they had let Clarke down, but more determined than ever to get it right and make the market work safely and sensibly. A few weeks later the message went out to regional managers to avoid radical changes to patient flows to hospitals in the first year. If Clarke had given ground at this meeting the internal market might never have come about and the history of the NHS might have been very different.

Mrs Thatcher's advisers had been right to be concerned. A market simulation exercise conducted in East Anglia in May 1990 involving many leading NHS managers and academics had collapsed.[161] The need for a market regulator to curb the worst excesses of an unfettered market was already clear.

Instead of simply creating NHS trusts, the Department of Health decided to invite local hospital managers to apply for trust status. In many cases they had to do so against the wishes of the health authorities that employed them. It was a time for bravery. It was the regional managers and their teams who persuaded many reluctant colleagues to apply, but it was the headquarters team in London that guided the volunteers through the process once the application had been lodged. In many hospitals staff took votes about the decision to apply. In practice, a large vote against by the doctors moved the application into the high-risk category.

Clarke and his colleagues fought the reform bill[364] through Parliament and it received Royal Assent on Friday 29 June 1990. The target date for implementation was 1 April 1991.

In October 1990 Nichol was able to report to the Policy Board in a 'state-of-readiness report' that 'there is now a general belief that services will be manageable through contracts in 1991/2.' The strong messages about smooth take-off and no surprises had been acted upon. Kenneth Clarke was very bullish about the progress that had been made, and expressed 'high confidence over the implementation of the reforms.'[163] 'Medical opposition was,' he thought, 'diminishing', and the first tranche of the promised 100 new consultant posts had been announced (all but one of these new posts were allocated to the surgical specialties). Work was beginning on the emerging strategic framework for the NHS.[164]

What was not clear to anybody, including Nichol, was how far the market would be allowed to develop. It was fine to use the market to 'put salt on the tails of those who did not perform',[147] but what if the competitive forces rendered a hospital non-viable? Could it be allowed to close, or would it have to be rescued? It was good to use the transparency of the market to expose poor clinical performance, but then what? Once the market got into full swing, could it be controlled or regulated? How to manage a market, once launched, even an internal one, became an important policy question.

The first steps in the creation of trusts (or self-governing hospitals as they were called at this stage) were taken in March 1989, when regional health authorities were asked to identify potential applicants.[165] There were only a few essential criteria:

- competent management with the commitment to apply
- adequate information systems
- senior professional staff involved in management
- financial viability
- not an escape from an unpalatable but necessary closure.

Staff ballots were considered but ruled out by Kenneth Clarke: 'No management issue in the NHS has ever been decided by ballot – not even the establishment of the NHS itself.'[166]

The policy of seeking volunteers for trust status and fundholding, rather than simply creating them by dictate in the manner of all previous reforms, was typical of Clarke. He valued the competition that this created, and was prepared to live with the controversy and conflict which it generated. Virginia Bottomley, who did not at all like the language of the market being used in health, thought this aspect of the reform management to be inspired. 'Trusts had to fight their corner and break through.'[167] She preferred to keep both fundholders and non-fundholders on the grounds that the improvements made in one group would inspire the other: 'This would keep both groups on their toes.'[167]

Nichol took a similar view, arguing that he saw the reforms as a developmental process and not a piece of administrative legislation. 'There were few managers with the capacity to handle what we meant by trust status. We could have changed the name on the outside of the hospital, but nothing much else would have changed.'[147]

The preparations continued with heightened urgency. All over the NHS, managers, doctors and all the other health professionals were consumed with the preparations for change. This time the Department of Health did not have a blueprint with all of the answers. Many problems had to be worked out on the ground. 'The NHS was about to go through a major metamorphism,' said Mike Malone Lee, the Director of Operations, but 'it could not leap straight away into new management arrangements and ways of working. There would be a transitional stage.'[168] He was wrong. The changes generated a momentum of their own as more trusts and fundholders than expected were ready at the start. It was a helter-skelter into the market. The best the centre could do was slow things down a little on the grounds of securing a safe take-off. The idea of a ' steady state' in the first year had never suited Clarke, who judged that there was little point in going through all the pain if there was to be no gain.

The definition of an acceptable trust took some time to emerge clearly. Huge acute hospital mergers, which would inhibit competition, were quickly ruled out, but proposals for whole district trusts (i.e. all services) in rural areas proved to be more difficult to resolve. Few were approved.

Community units were allowed to apply after the first round. The concept of 'core services' developed, which every District General Hospital would have to supply whether they wanted to or not. No one wanted hospitals to concentrate simply on profitable clinical practice.

In July 1990 the reconstituted regional health authorities came into being, followed in September by 190 reconstituted district health authorities and 90 family health service authorities. They had an entirely new constitution, with paid NHS employees becoming executive directors on their boards. It looked and felt more like a large business than a traditional public service.

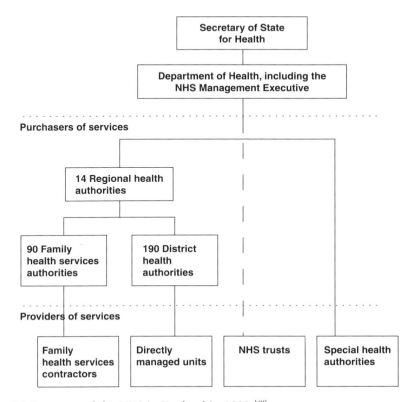

Figure 4.1 Structure of the NHS in England in 1990.[109]

With the benefit of hindsight, it later became clear that many DHAs had failed to develop the purchasing agenda with the energy and vision that were required. Many chief executives and their authorities grieved about the potential loss of the directly managed units as they changed to trust status. Some chief executives were not at all sure of what their new role would be once they had lost their hospital and community units. Such a view was, in the eyes of Chris Spry, the RGM who led the national team focused on purchasing 'Naive – it overlooked the need for balance between the longer-term vision of healthcare for the local district, public and political expectations and what was realistic. These judgements were the territory of the District General Manager.'[169] In practice, DHAs had to set up Chinese walls between those parts of their organisation that were responsible for purchasing and those that were still in charge of provider units and services. 'Holding on but letting go' became the catchphrase.[170] The new FHSAs had a clearer agenda, to promote fundholding and introduce Indicative Prescribing Budgets, which were intended to start the process of capping drug expenditure at a local level.

Waldegrave takes over

In November 1990 Kenneth Clarke, with just four months to go before the launch of the reforms, moved to the Department of Education and William Waldegrave took over as Secretary of State. His brief from Mrs Thatcher was clear: 'Kenneth has made all the changes and stirred them up, and you have got to quieten things down.'[171] He received an upbeat report from Nichol on the state of readiness of the NHS to enter the internal market. During the preceding months the Executive had undertaken a series of regional stock takes which had confirmed 'the tremendous progress that had been made.' A smooth take-off looked to be assured. This was true for much of the country.

However, there were black spots where progress had been slow and where it was proving very difficult to reconcile the cash that purchasers had available to spend with the sums that provider units expected to let them have to balance their books. London as always was proving particularly challenging. The announcement of 600 redundancies at Guy's Hospital in London by Peter Griffiths, the former deputy NHS Chief Executive, caused a storm.[172] Even more worrying was Nichol's briefing on bed closures, which had been in the headlines as a result of a report compiled by the National Association of Health Authorities and Trusts (NAHAT) predicting 3000 bed closures. Nichol thought that this was an underestimate. As the CMO put it during this briefing, 'the system was very stretched.'[173]

William Waldegrave, Secretary of State, 1990–92

William Waldegrave was educated at Eton, Corpus Christi College, Oxford and Harvard University. His working career has included the Civil Service, industry, farming in the West Country, and acting as a general adviser in the Cabinet Office.

He became MP for Bristol West in 1979. Between 1981 and 1985 he was Parliamentary Under-Secretary of State in Education and Science and in the

Department of the Environment. He was later Minister of State in both the Department of the Environment and the Foreign Office. He was Secretary of State for Health from 1990 to 1992. He later held ministerial posts in Public Service and Science, Agriculture, Fisheries and Food, and the Treasury.

The doctors sought to establish an *entente cordiale* with the new Secretary of State. Waldegrave listened to them carefully but was not prepared to budge an inch on the principle of introducing competition into the NHS. 'The NHS embodies an ideal,' he told the Tory Party Central Committee in March 1991, 'but this does not mean we should not subject its ramshackle structures, jerry-built in the 1940s and clad in concrete in the 1960s, to the most rigorous appraisal'.[174] However, he did try to change the language and he re-emphasised that comparing cost and performance was very important in the public services. On a number of occasions he reiterated the Government's commitment to the NHS. 'The issue is not whether we have an NHS, but what the nature of that service should be and how it is organised. We are all equal in the face of death,' he told the party faithful, 'access to the same healthcare united duke and dustman in 1948 as members of the same national family. It unites their successors still.' He was also clear that the NHS was going to remain a public service. The changes were, he said, 'aimed at the production of an efficient public service, funded by public money.'[174]

Virginia Bottomley, his Minister of State, reinforced his message in her own way and sought to fit the market into public service principles: 'As a former public sector person myself, the commercial language of the market was as alien to me as it was to most people in the NHS.'[167]

Waldegrave extended the membership of the Policy Board in 1991 to include Peter Gummer and Jean Denton, both experts in public relations. Anne Poole, the CNO, had joined the Board 'on a renewal basis' in November 1990, which was technically at least the same basis as that on which the CMO had been appointed earlier.[175] The market went live in April 1991. Eventually 57 hospitals got through to trust status (far more than Clarke had anticipated) and attended a private celebratory dinner at the Banqueting House, much to the disquiet of Virginia Bottomley, who thought such ostentatious celebration inappropriate.[167]

GP fundholding followed pretty much the same pattern. Volunteers had been sought, and enough were forthcoming to ensure a satisfactory launch, with 306 practices by 1 April 1991. At this stage their budgets were very provisional indeed. The early fundholding practices embraced the idea with evangelical zeal. They revelled in the power it gave them over the consultants. GPs suddenly had authority and influence and they rather liked it. Their enthusiasm took much of the wind out of the sails of the BMA, which continued to argue against their existence. The BMA opposition to NHS trusts was similarly blunted by the majority of hospital doctors, who welcomed their institutions' newfound freedom.

The notion that patients in fundholding practices were receiving preferential access to hospital services (the two-tier debate) had proved troublesome from the start. It was certainly true that some fundholders had negotiated speedy access for their patients. It was one of the service improvements that they most wanted to secure. The BMA and the Opposition attacked hard on this point. The NHS had to serve everybody, not just a few.

In June 1991, Waldegrave and Nichol took much of the steam out of the argument with an agreement with the Joint Consultants Committee and the General Medical Services Committee about the operation of the market. Hospitals were told to ensure that their doctors were more closely involved in negotiating contracts, and were not to offer deals to one purchaser that would disadvantage the patients of another. The decision about who to treat and when was to be made on the basis of clinical need, and must be made by the hospital consultant. Common waiting lists were to be introduced for urgent and seriously ill patients and for those waiting for highly specialised treatments.[176] However, the agreement did confirm that GPs could if they wished refer patients to a consultant for an opinion only, leaving them and their patient to decide whether to accept the consultant's advice about treatment. Fundholders were told not to impose unreasonable quality standards on providers, and hospitals were told to stop cost shifting by varying the apportionment of overheads.

It was now clear to all that the NHS was operating in a managed market, not a free for all. The competitive games and the aggression that had been evident in the early stages had to stop. There were rules, procedures and ethics, and they had to be followed.

Sheila Masters

Sheila Masters was a partner in Peat, Marwick and Mitchell when she was seconded to be Director of Finance on the NHS Management Executive, 1979–81. She is now Baroness Noakes. She was Director of the Bank of England 1994–2000 and has held many directorships in the commercial sector.

In July 1991, Waldegrave and Nichol made preparations for a report to John Major, now the Prime Minister. They rehearsed it a number of times with the help of Peter Gummer, the new Policy Board member. They reported that the structure of the reformed NHS was in place and money was being distributed to district health authorities to purchase services for their local communities. There remained some disparity in the per capita allocations, which would be evened out in a year or two.

NHS contracts were in place between health authorities (purchasers) and trusts (providers), and although the first batch of contracts were relatively simple, and reflected the status quo, many included some quality standards.

Nichol reported that the trust movement was growing fast and that the first wave was doing well. Fundholding had got off to a fine start and covered 7% of the population. On the finance side, about which John Major knew quite a lot from his days at the Treasury, the news was also good. The NHS was paying its bills on time, and deficits had been largely driven out of the system. Waiting lists had started to fall, with large reductions in the numbers waiting for over a year. The only real problem on the horizon was the possibility that some hospitals would fail to manage their workload to fit within their block contract, particularly in London.

The number of patients being treated was rising, which was important because any significant drop in the number of patients being treated would have led to serious difficulties with the Treasury.

Sheila Master's presentation to the Prime Minister on the financial outlook, 1991–92[177]

Good news	*Pressure points*
More patients being treated (2% growth or more)	Extra-contractual referrals (1.3%)
Fewer long waiting times	Danger of stop/start in winter
Deficits gone	Slow-down in new capital schemes
Creditors being paid off	Demands from trusts for more income
Block contracts (97%)	
Standby (0.4% for risk)	
Inflation (0.3% cushion)	

Waldegrave and Nichol were very upbeat about the future at this meeting with John Major. Fair funding for purchasers would be in place by 1995–96, future contracts would have more and more quality requirements, and there would be many more fundholders to challenge the traditional boundaries between primary and secondary care. All hospitals would become trusts within three years. The principal risk in moving forward from the 'steady state' would be seen most clearly in London, which had poor primary care, a concentration of teaching facilities and 1000 too many beds.

Now that the reform infrastructure was in place, it needed time for 'polishing off the rough edges'. 'The door,' Waldegrave and Nichol explained, 'was just opening'. More and more staff, they reported, were beginning to see opportunities in the new arrangements. It was a process of 'levelling up standards in order to achieve greater equity at a higher level.' They used, by way of example, the work in the Mersey region to tackle waiting lists and particularly to offer treatment to those at the end of the longest lists.

The timetable of future events, which was a backcloth to these discussions, was presented as follows:

1991

July	Launch of Patient's Charter (to be built into 1992–93 contracts)
End September	DHA purchasing plans for 1992–93 available Expect noise from losing trusts
Early October	Decisions about second-wave trusts
November	Second quarter monitoring information available which will show performance against plan for first six months
Autumn	Financial Statement
December	Decisions about manageability of the 1992–93 plans

1992	
February	Third quarter monitoring information available
	Purchasers to get confirmation about allocations
March	Second-wave fundholders determined.

At the 1991 Conservative Party Conference, John Major responded to continuing challenges from the Labour Party about creeping privatisation by declaring that there would be 'no privatisation of healthcare, neither piecemeal, nor in part, nor in whole, not today, not tomorrow, not after the next election, not ever, whilst I am Prime Minister.' Health was still a hot political issue.

Attempts to communicate the message that the reforms would enhance the reputation of the NHS were a recurrent managerial and political theme during this period. For the most part the Department and the Executive were losing the communications battle. Bad news always drove out good. Uncertainty created confusion. In October 1991, the Policy Board returned to the Burson Marsteller/ Kingsley Lord communications work, first commissioned in 1989, which had surveyed communication practices and staff attitudes in the NHS nationwide. It was a large survey covering a quarter of a million people, and it had confirmed what everybody knew. Staff neither understood nor welcomed the reforms, and this included many of their managers.[178] Nichol had undertaken a whistle-stop tour of the country in the early part of 1990 in an attempt to improve matters, but the impact had been minimal. Steps were now urgently needed to refocus the message and co-ordinate the public relations effort at the centre with that in the field. Gummer's advice to Waldegrave was that 'we must as a Board be able to ensure that our employees and market are neither misled nor ill-informed.' He recommended that a communications team be appointed, with delegated responsibility, a budget and personnel, who would be told to get on with the job.[179]

One result was the decision to let the NHS Executive launch its own annual report. It came out in November 1992 with a front cover that stated 'We are the largest employer in Europe, with a workforce of over 850 000, with a turnover in excess of £26 billion and serving a community of 47 million people. We share one aim.' On page two was the aim – 'to create a better health service for the nation.' The Executive was taking the battle to the media.[180]

Nichol's relationship with John Major as Prime Minister was focused primarily on the introduction of *The Patient's Charter* into the NHS, and on changes to the NHS in London. Major took a close interest in the impact of the reforms in London.

One of the most contentious of all the new trust freedoms was the ability to settle pay locally. The policy objective was to introduce more flexibility into the rigid framework of national pay so that local managers could relate pay rates to local labour markets and reward individual performance. A modest step had been taken in 1969, which allowed local managers to make supplements to national scales for administrative and clerical staff where there were difficulties with regard to recruitment and retention. The following year this was extended to cover scientific, professional and technical staff, and a pilot scheme began with nurses and midwives. The ambulance settlement had also had an element of local flexibility built into it. The number of staff covered by national agreements was expected to fall sharply and thus reduce the influence of the Whitley system of pay bargaining. The trade unions strongly opposed these moves. Despite much encouragement from the centre, most trusts elected to adhere initially to the national agreements. However, Eric Caines, the new Director of Personnel, was pushed hard for more progress and actively encouraged NHS managers to grasp the nettle and use their new powers. Duncan Nichol was more cautious and insisted on a managed and orderly programme of change. He had judged the mood of the trusts correctly. Most of them were busy enough as it was without having to find time for a fight with the unions. In any case there remained significant doubts within the Department of Health about the capacity of some managers to handle local negotiation. The Department sought to reduce the flow of questions from the NHS about the interpretation of national agreements. Sometimes these questions were legitimate, but often the Department was being asked to referee a turf battle between the personnel and the payroll departments, who wanted to be absolutely sure that they could not be criticised by the auditors. NHS management, the Executive argued, must learn to stand on its own feet and make its own judgements. They represented the employers, not the Department of Health.

However, Caines' pressure was to have an unplanned consequence as some managers began to make local decisions and ignore the established rules. Many of the decisions they took, especially those with regard to termination settlements, were technically beyond their powers and needed a specific authorisation by the Secretary of State, called a variation order. Whatever officials said, the auditors would later insist that the rules should have been followed to the letter.

The structure of the NHS was at this point still fluid. The Management Executive for England had been established and reported to a Policy Board, chaired by the Secretary of State. The Policy Board was supposed to hold the Executive to account, but never really did. The strategic goals set for the Executive in 1991–92 ran to 12 pages and covered everything from grand strategy to specific targets such as the requirement that no patient should wait longer than 24 months for non-urgent surgery. The flow of information between the Executive and the Policy Board had been carefully negotiated behind the scenes in order to ensure that the Policy Board did not meddle in the day-to-day affairs of the NHS, but it often did.

The increasing sophistication of the Executive meetings is demonstrated by the allocation in April 1992 of a whole day to agreeing how to integrate research and development into the mainstream management agenda.

The Executive and the Region: the Waldegrave letter

Regions still took the lead role in implementing the reforms on the ground, but they wanted oversight of the new trusts. Oversight was the most they could expect, as the chairmen of trusts and their boards were accountable directly to the Secretary of State who appointed them. It was denied them, and the trusts continued to report directly to the Department of Health through their newly created network of outposts (much to the delight of the trusts, which preferred their 'light touch' approach that focused almost entirely on finance). The regional chairmen kept pushing the point. They had got on well with Fowler and Clarke and continued to think of themselves as the Secretary of State's NHS Cabinet, which could handle both the politics and the management of the NHS. They had created their own secretariat in London and saw themselves as sitting alongside the NHS Executive (and certainly not reporting to it) and able to offer support. However, they did retain their right to offer different advice to ministers if they thought this necessary. The regional managers, led by their chairman Brian Edwards, had started to dismantle their own separate meetings and working groups and to move with Nichol towards single-centre working. The Executive and the regional managers began to meet on a monthly basis. Nichol usually attended the private meetings of regional chairmen, who continued to have regular meetings with the Secretary of State. Handling these complex relationships consumed a great deal of Nichol's time and energies.

An analysis of the business of these various groups showed substantial overlap. As Chris France explained:

> The Thatcher Review did not seize on one of the central dilemmas of the NHS, which was whether it was centrally or regionally managed. The regional health authorities survived. I think this was largely a political decision. They were stuffed to the gunwales with Tories and we know they were influential locally. Don Wilson, Chairman of the Mersey Region, was the quintessential example of this. He was a great fixer and deliverer of things locally, and ministers did not want to lose that, and they did not want to put noses out of joint and remove people like Don Wilson out of high-profile jobs. They kept the regional health authorities and increased the profile of the Management Executive. An important structural issue had been dodged. Regional chairmen continued to report to ministers and regional managers to their boards. Ministers wanted it both ways and relied on all the parties working together.[120]

Waldegrave valued his relationship with the regional chairmen, whom he regarded 'as part of the political team running the NHS with ministers',[181] but would not give way on the question of trust accountability. Eventually he wrote formally to Sir Donald Wilson after a meeting with him on 6 March 1991. Eric Caines and the Trust Unit in the Department drafted the letter.

> Trusts will not be accountable to regions but to me and my successors as Secretary of State. The Management Executive will monitor the performance of trusts on my behalf. Regions will work through the purchasing line to ensure that contracts, which are placed with trusts, are designed to achieve national healthcare priorities as well as reflect local needs. Regions will not be expected to manage the market by dictating that trusts should or should not provide particular services, except in the case of designated services. The risks attendant upon a change in the pattern of service provision will be for trusts to take.[182]

The Trust Unit was determined to keep the regional health authorities (or the 'dinosaurs', as they referred to them) at bay. They and others in the Department worried that the regional health authorities would stifle innovation and development even though they had borne the brunt of the task of implementing the internal market. The centre was getting increasingly uncomfortable with the tendency of some regions to take an independent line on key policy issues and particularly the pace of change.

Waldegrave's letter represented a sharp rebuff for the regional chairmen in particular, and from this point on their role and influence began to diminish. Ministers and Nichol began to think through what a single centre would look like, and this led on to discussions about a new intermediate tier. Waldegrave had also shifted his view about the regions, which he now regarded as a rival management structure to the Executive. If he had stayed in office much longer he would have disbanded them earlier than was the case.[181]

In September 1991 Sheila Masters had produced for the Executive a league table of regional performance. It was based on a number of criteria, including the 1990–91 financial outcome, the quality and timeliness of information that they had provided, the quality of their 1991–92 plans and the number of Directly Managed Units that were in trouble.[179] (Directly Managed Units were those hospitals and community units that had not yet achieved trust status and were thus still accountable to DHAs and the regions.)

Chris France blocked the publication of the table, on the grounds that he did not understand the underlying logic, but it leaked into the system and caused much comment at regional meetings. The Department of Health was later to make extensive use of such tables as a stimulus to performance. The tables added to Sheila Masters' reputation as a tough customer, and showed that the Executive was serious in its intention to oversee the performance of the regional health authorities.

Sheila Masters' table: who is doing OK in 1991–92[179]

Maximum score = +5   Minimum score = −5

1	+3	West Midlands
2	+3	South Western
3	+2	North Western
4	+1	Trent
5	+1	South West Thames
6	0	Yorkshire
7	0	Wessex
8	0	Oxford
9	−1	East Anglia
9	−1	Mersey
10	−2	Northern
11	−4	North West Thames
12	−4	North East Thames
13	−5	South East Thames

Health of the Nation

The territory upon which Waldegrave found common ground with the doctors was the production of a new plan based on health rather than economic foundations. It was *Health of the Nation*.[138] Preparations had begun during Clarke's term of office with ideas about national strategic frameworks and performance measurement. Some health authorities had produced their own 'health gain targets' following the publication of the World Health Organization plan *Health for All in the Year 2000*.[373] Under Waldegrave the plan developed into a full-scale health strategy. Both the Executive and the Policy Divisions worked on this subject and the CMO personally played a major part. It was a good example of the wider Department of Health working together. Waldegrave saw it as an opportunity to create a 'rational underpinning for policy as well as a way of reuniting the health community.'[181] John Major invited all the major NHS players to a meeting at Chequers to work through the principles and build up some commitment to implementation. Leading managers mixed with presidents of Royal Colleges, the NHS Executive and a full ministerial team. The meeting had a relaxed atmosphere and went well, despite some tough talking by the doctors about tobacco advertising. It was agreed at this meeting that some choices would have to be made. Everything could not be a priority.

The Patient's Charter

The growing interest in and concern with quality had been stimulated by the launch of the health version of the Citizen's Charter. With the Prime Minister driving it, this policy moved in Whitehall. Duncan Nichol created a special task group, which toured the country promoting the policy and checking on its implementation.[137] Soon copies of the Charter began to appear in hospitals all over the country, and for the first time patients had explicit standards against which to judge the service they had received. Many patients, and their carers, started to take advantage of their rights, much to the discomfort of some professionals.

The Patient's Charter 1991[137]

Patients' Rights

1 To receive healthcare on the basis of clinical need, regardless of the ability to pay.
2 To be registered with a GP.
3 To receive emergency medical care at any time through a GP or through the emergency ambulance service and a hospital Accident and Emergency department.
4 To be referred to a consultant, acceptable to the patient, when a GP thinks this is necessary, and to be referred for a second opinion if a patient and the GP agree this to be desirable.
5 To be given a clear explanation of any treatment proposed, including any risk or alternatives.
6 To have access to health records, and to know that those working in the NHS are under a legal duty to keep their contents confidential.
7 To choose whether or not to take part in medical research or medical student training.

8 To be given detailed information on local health services, including quality standards and maximum waiting times.

9 To be guaranteed admission for treatment by a specific date no more than two years from the day the patient was put on the waiting list.

10 To have any complaint about NHS services investigated, and to receive a full and prompt written reply from the Chief Executive concerned.

Most of these rights already existed, of course, but presenting them in this way was to have a powerful impact on the NHS. Most thought the impact was good, but some warned about unreasonable citizens who would abuse such rights. Patients also have duties and obligations, they argued. The first set of standards was very hospital focused, and later versions (of which there were many) included primary care and mental health. Later governments were to crank up the standards for access to non-acute care.

Parliamentary accountability

In 1990, Nichol made his first appearance before a Committee of the House of Commons. It was the first of seven appearances in the next two years. The toughest committee to appear before was undoubtedly the Public Accounts Committee (PAC), which was chaired, from June 1992, by Robert Sheldon. Nichol appeared as the Accounting Officer for the NHS budget in England. The Social Services Select Committee, with Nicholas Winterton in the chair, could also be tough once they got their teeth into an issue.

The preparations for an appearance began well in advance with a prodigious amount of briefing, all of which had to be mastered and assimilated before the day of the appearance. A colleague sometimes accompanied Nichol, but the civil servants who had handled the preparation of the brief had to secure a seat in the public gallery immediately behind him. The questioning was tough and sometimes politically partisan. There were unspoken conventions and rules. Although one could hold a line if one believed in it, it rarely paid off to take the offensive. Nichol was expected to have the detail at his fingertips, a task that was clearly impossible given the huge range of subjects about which he was questioned, ranging from capital developments to cervical cytology. It was his memory that was being tested, not his judgement. On one occasion he railed against a series of detailed questions about the Pearce Inquiry into services for the younger disabled. 'I do not see the job as counting aniseed balls in a jam jar in the corner shop.' 'So,' said the MP, 'let us return to younger, disabled aniseed balls. You are obviously not well briefed.' 'Not at all,' said Nichol, 'No, it is not a question of not being well briefed. I just do not see the point in this.' 'Well, how many people have you got behind you?' asked the MP. 'About a dozen,' said Nichol. 'Well, do they know anything?' 'We could ask them,' Nichol replied. It was not at all amusing.[147]

Nichol raised these matters with John Bourn, Comptroller and Auditor General and head of the National Audit Office, and out of that conversation began the moves that would result in trust chief executives being made accounting officers as well. This reflected a broader move across Whitehall which had been prompted by the need to make the heads of lower-level entities, who now headed Next

Steps Agencies, accounting officers and thereby eligible to be called before the PAC.

Two subjects caused Nichol the most concern, and none had much to do with decisions he had made himself. The first was a Regional Information Systems Development Plan (RISP) in Wessex that had gone seriously wrong. There had been cost overruns, delays and, crucially, a loss of faith in the developing system by users. When the plug was finally pulled on the scheme the losses were conservatively assessed at around £20 million. Allegations about conflicts of interest by some of the parties involved added to the problems. The Department of Health got its knuckles rapped for not intervening earlier than it did.

The second issue was to do with problems in the West Midlands Region, which largely centred on a programme of dis-investments in a wide range of regional services, including estates, computing and supplies. The audit criticisms were focused on contracts, guarantees and loans placed without proper sanction by officers of the Authority. As the PAC put it, 'a responsible official, new to the NHS, was able to follow his own path, making a bonfire of the rules in the process, uncontrolled by either the RHA or senior regional management.'[188] QA Business Services, the company created by the floating off of the former management services division, collapsed quite quickly, leaving former public service staff with sharply reduced pensions. According to the PAC there had been 'a serious failure by the member of the Regional Authority, and in particular the Chairman, in their duty to secure the accountability of regional management.'[188]

However, this was not all that was wrong in Birmingham. A major plan to rationalise the hospitals in the city had come under fire from the City Council and the local press. By May 1994, the Birmingham Health Authorities were slipping into a major financial crisis that had reached £16 million, following a messy merger of the South Birmingham and Central Birmingham health authorities in April 1991. The handling of these problems at the Department by the Executive was complicated by the fact that the regional chairman, James Ackers, was a powerful national figure with a seat on the Policy Board who also had close contacts with ministers. He played the role of an executive chairman in his own Region with a very hands-on approach. To complicate matters yet further, his personal circumstances were in disarray. His family business had gone bust, and this had affected him deeply. Now his NHS world was in crisis. Eventually, far later than should have been the case, he was forced to resign and a new team was drafted in to clear up the mess. First Don Wilson, the Mersey Chairman and by far the most senior and influential of the regional chairmen, took over on a temporary basis and set about re-establishing the confidence of the local politicians and the press. With every Board meeting surrounded by the media looking to build up the crisis it was a tough assignment, but within a few months Wilson had settled things down. Brian Edwards, the RGM from Trent, was persuaded by Nichol to move across to Birmingham to continue his work with a new chairman, Bryan Baker. Together they sorted out the troubled West Midlands, and Birmingham itself slowly and painfully climbed out of crisis. The move of senior people between regions had never occurred before, and this gave another signal about the growing power and confidence of the Executive.

It was Baker and Edwards who had to accompany Nichol to a highly charged Public Accounts Committee hearing in February 1994 to explain what had gone wrong and what was being done to sort out the mess.[183]

In both the Wessex and West Midlands cases the auditors had strongly attacked what they regarded as improper, unauthorised and over-generous termination payments for senior staff. The absence of variation orders, which would have legitimised such payments, came home to roost.

The pressure over this issue eventually became so great that Nichol insisted all regions came clean about any termination payments that had been made (known as the Venning Trawl, after the name of the officer in charge), so that retrospective authority to make them could be sought from the Treasury. There were many red faces and more than a few managers who worried about their professional futures.

Nichol was to become a powerful performer in front of parliamentary committees, but this absorbed an enormous amount of his time at the expense of his day-to-day engagement with the NHS.

The *Daily Mail* affair

In October 1991, William Waldegrave asked Duncan Nichol to do an interview with a journalist from the *Daily Mail*.[147] For weeks the media had been attacking the Government and suggesting that the Tories were intent on privatising the NHS. It had all started with a vigorous speech by Neil Kinnock at the Labour Party Conference. 'Labour,' he said, 'want to strengthen the NHS and ensure that it survives as a people's service, in stark contrast to the Tories, who want to take it to pieces, to make it a creature of contracts and commerce.' The slogan 'Only vote Conservative if you want the Health Service destroyed' was a powerful one. Even Mrs Thatcher was worried when she was told about the effect of this speech on the election polls, and she instructed her team that was writing the manifesto to ensure it included a promise that the NHS would not be privatised.

Nichol had good reason to be concerned about what the Labour team was up to. Some MPs had made it very plain to managers who were leading bids for trust status that they had no personal future in the NHS should Labour return to office. It was straightforward intimidation that Robin Cook, then opposition spokesman on health, chose to ignore rather than deny.

Nichol agreed to do an interview although he knew that an election was close. On this occasion he did not engage his press office or have a minder with him. (The NHS Executive had its own communications team.) He for one did not want the NHS privatised, and he had no evidence that ministers did either. He said as much in blunt and unequivocal terms. 'There was not a shred of evidence,' he said, 'that the Government were intent on privatising the NHS.'[184]

This was strong stuff, and Robin Cook was furious. He demanded a retraction and an apology from Sir Robin Butler, the head of the Civil Service. 'It was,' he said, 'dangerous for ministers to be seen to be putting the Civil Service in the front of controversy, and was damaging to the Service's impartiality.'[185] Nichol was summoned to see Butler, who then took the lead with Chris France in preparing a response to Cook. They regarded this as a very serious matter, as Nichol was judged to have crossed an important line in the relationship between civil servants and politicians. Nichol was actively supporting one side of the political divide against the other.[186] Nichol of course saw it differently, and said so. 'We are not trying to privatise the NHS,' he told them. 'If we were, I am conniving at it and fooling a lot of people in the NHS and that's one thing I am not going to do. I might be stupid and they [the politicians] are pulling the wool over my eyes, but I don't think that is true either.'[147]

Drafts of a response to Cook flew across Whitehall. The first draft sounded to Nichol very much like an apology, and he said as much. A second draft was dispatched up to John Major in Blackpool, where the Conservative Party was holding its conference. Major did not like it, and insisted that the reply should support Nichol. Eventually a compromise was struck whereby Butler assured Cook that there had been no 'intentional overstepping the mark.'

Nichol received strong public support from the Prime Minister, but what Nichol did not know was that his fellow permanent secretaries were in revolt. This was a 'politicised civil servant' in action and it was dangerous. It opened the door to the idea that senior civil servants could come and go with changes of government. First Division (the association that represents senior civil servants) piled in with their own press statement accusing Nichol of going beyond the bounds of political neutrality. 'It appears in this particular case that the statement has gone beyond the point of explaining Government policy to the point of actually promoting Government policy and then attacking the opposition.'[186] What Robin Butler needed to say, but did not, was that in the modern world there were different types of permanent secretary. Some were intelligent, thoughtful and entirely neutral policy advisers. Others, in order to be successful, had to believe in what they were doing with a passion and take others with them. Nichol was not neutral about the NHS reforms. He believed in them. If they had been reversed in his time he would have resigned.

Waldegrave thought that Nichol was entirely within his rights to give the interview but was aware, at least on reflection, that it did indeed represent a challenge to the tradition of neutrality. He explains:

> When Harold Wilson walked into Downing Street all the private secretaries who had worked for Edward Heath were clapping as he came through the door. The Constitution was working perfectly. Civil servants have to be chameleons and they have to do as their ministers tell them. Managers, on the other hand, have to commit to and own a management plan.[181]

Nichol was being urged by his own instincts and by ministers to speak out in support of what he was trying to achieve. He was following the brief given to him by Mrs Thatcher to be a visible leader.

The matter died, but Nichol strongly suspected that his chances of survival would be slim if Robin Cook ever became Secretary of State for Health.

Nichol's stand produced a mixed reaction among NHS managers. For many who were tired of their efforts to reform the system being constantly denigrated in the press, it was a timely intervention. For others it was, according to the *Health Services Journal*, a disaster:

> So long as Mr Nichol maintained a scrupulous distance from party politics, he acted as a shield for all managers. The danger in abandoning his neutrality is that he has given substance to the belief that some managers are biased politically and create a climate in which it would be easier for a Labour Government to remove them.[187]

There is no doubt that Nichol's stand damaged him in Whitehall. When the time came for a knighthood it was blocked until Bottomley intervened and insisted that it went through. This question of how close a chief executive could get to his ministers is of crucial importance. With Clarke, Waldegrave and Bottomley, Nichol was very much part of their kitchen cabinet. He attended meetings of high political sensitivity but kept his political views to himself. When matters got very political Nichol was, according to Waldegrave, very good at leaving the room.[181]

In April 1992, John Major won the general election and Virginia Bottomley became Secretary of State for Health with Brian Mawhinney as Minister of Health. William Waldegrave moved on to the Cabinet Office and Kenneth Clarke became Home Secretary. Graham Hart had returned from Scotland to take up the post of Permanent Secretary in January.

Virginia Bottomley takes over as Secretary of State

At this point the organisation of the Department was as shown in Figure 4.2. Virginia Bottomley was surprised and delighted with her promotion, which was welcomed by Nichol and his team, who had developed a good working relationship with her. She could be frustrating and she liked to circle difficult decisions, taking soundings from many sources, rather than dealing with them directly. She also listened assiduously to the early-morning edition of the *Today* programme on the radio, and demanded immediate answers and responses to any critical health stories. She believed in the NHS and had a natural sympathy with its purpose. She knew personally many of the big players in the health world. Although her first instincts had been against the market in healthcare, she had undergone a complete conversion when 'I realised that this rather unattractive business-school language was really about a profound change in the balance of power which I, as a former sociologist, entirely endorsed. It would move the power from the institutions to the agents of the people.'[167]

The reform programme continued, but with a softer media image and an easier relationship with the health professions. An early priority was to energise the purchasing end of the market and get beyond a simple block contract for a poorly defined set of services at a fixed total price. This left all the pressure and risks on the provider units and trusts in particular. DHAs were themselves in a state of constant change, which undoubtedly slowed down their role development. By March 1994 there had been 44 mergers, and more were forecast for April 1995. Bottomley left Brian Mawhinney with the task of energising the purchasers, with Nichol's support. They had some success, which led the *British Medical Journal* to refer to purchasers as 'big and ugly', which most took to be a compliment.

The two-tier argument continued to bedevil the fundholding movement, and it was true that good fundholding practices could and sometimes did secure more timely treatment for their patients. The range of services included within the budget had gradually expanded, and in a few cases successful practices were allowed to go the whole hog and become what was termed *total fundholders* (i.e. they were given all the money to purchase all services for their patients). This was a development that started in the field with sympathetic regions, rather than as a result of a national policy decision.

In Bromsgrove, a market town in Worcestershire, the four practices in the town

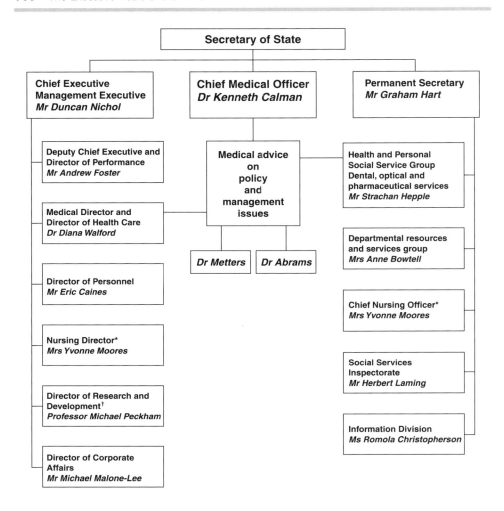

*Mrs Moores had a dual role as CNO of the Department and Nursing Director of the NHS Management Executive.

†Professor Peckham was responsible for Research and Development for the Department as a whole as well as for the NHS Management Executive.

Figure 4.2 Structure of the Department of Health in 1992.

had been early fundholders. They had worked well together and negotiated with providers as a team. In 1993 they teamed up with two more practices in a neighbouring town to create a single negotiating unit with a common set of contracts. By April 1994 they were ready to take on the contracting for all services for their community. The first total fundholding scheme was launched. An independent evaluation published in 1997 confirmed that local purchasing had produced significant benefits, but it had not been easy. Sorting out the relationships between the staff working directly for the GPs and those employed by the Community Trust had been difficult, but forcing change in the acute hospital sector had been really tough.[189]

GPs with a fundamental objection to fundholding began to work as commissioning groups with their local health authorities. It was becoming complicated, but interesting, as the early pioneers broke new ground. Soon, though, financial holes began to appear in the budgets of some fundholding practices. They argued, of course, that the budget was inadequate, and in some cases they were right. However, in other cases it was down to incompetence, and action had to be taken, albeit with great reluctance, to remove fundholder status from some practices. The brave experiment was taking on a harder edge.

The *Health of the Nation* plan,[138] when it was published in July 1992, targeted five key areas, namely coronary heart disease, cancer, HIV/AIDS, mental health and accidents. This was a very important development and, as *The Times* put it, 'took the Department of Health and the NHS beyond a healthcare service to health itself.' It was also an important point in the re-establishment of working relations between the Government and the professions. Although the policy worked in the sense that many of the targets were achieved, it did not survive the passage of time, and quietly faded from the scene after some initial revamping by the next Government. By 1997 its impact on local decision making was negligible.[190] Some would argue that it had been successfully assimilated into the system of government and the core of NHS policy. A more sanguine view is that all political initiatives in health have a sell-by date. In any case, as Frank Dobson was later to express it, 'it was good at making people in Surrey healthier, but it was not making much impact on Hackney.'[191]

However, the management agenda inside the Department of Health was moving far more decisively into public health and clinical territories. The CMO made a number of important contributions to both the Management Executive and the Policy Board during this period, introducing the Executive to the potential impact of clinical development in fields such as genetics, and keeping up the pressure on AIDS investment.

Public health policy was to return as a major issue in 2004 after ministers had decided to ask the public how far they should go in promoting anti-smoking and obesity programmes.

Move to Leeds

In July 1992 the Executive moved into new offices in Quarry House, Leeds. The decision to move the Executive out of London was taken by Ken Clarke on his final day in office as Secretary of State in November 1990.[181] He wanted to clear the desk for his successor. The move was part of a wider policy of dispersing government to the provinces, but had the added attraction to both Clarke and Nichol of creating physical distance between ministers and the Executive. This would, they judged, enable the Executive to develop a sharper and more distinctive image of its own. France, who had worked up the briefing paper for ministers, with Nichol and the CMO, was surprised by the decision. It did not accord with the official advice that Clarke had received.

> It was [France thought] based on two delusions. The first was Nichol's view that 'if the Executive moved to Leeds it would somehow be free of the political trammels of Whitehall.' The second was Clarke's view that the physical distance would enable him to legitimately deflect to Nichol detailed questions about the operation of the NHS, and when

things went wrong 'everyone would say it was the awful management in Leeds, not the Secretary of State in London.'[120]

Nichol and his senior team kept an office in London as well. Everybody had to be trained in video conferencing. Today almost everybody, including Nichol, regards the move as a mistake. The Executive moved, but the power and day-to-day decision making stayed in London with ministers. The irony is that it might never have happened. Waldegrave might never have agreed.

> I should have stopped it. It was a classic 'Yes Minister' thing. Not by the Civil Service on this occasion, but by one's predecessor. One should always look at decisions that have been taken in the last few days when someone knows they are going. I thought it a complete mistake, in that it was a theoretical step, which meant that everybody lived on trains. It was a waste of money and damaging and made life difficult for everybody.[181]

London

London was also in need of a solution and, as a London MP, Mrs Bottomley was very sensitive to its problems. London's population had decreased by 20% between 1979 and 1992, yet the average number of beds in the capital was 4.1 per 100 000 population, compared with 2.6 per 100 000 in the rest of England.[192] Patients in the Greater London area were increasingly going to their local hospital rather than to hospitals in the centre of the city. Many of the hospitals in central London needed urgent refurbishment and development. Primary care was very patchy indeed. A strategic development plan was needed. Bernard Tomlinson, a pathologist from Newcastle and former Regional Chairman in the North East, had been drafted in by Waldegrave in 1991 to undertake yet another London Hospitals review. He reported in October 1992.[139] He recommended major improvements in primary care via Primary Care Development Zones, and a major rationalisation of the hospital sector. Some of the large hospitals would have to merge (Guy's and St Thomas's. Bart's and the London). The specialist hospitals such as the Royal Brompton and Great Ormond Street would be better if they were integrated into larger units. (The London postgraduate hospitals had been excluded from the first years of the internal market and had retained their reserved funding streams, much to the envy of many other centres outside the capital.) Bottomley accepted most of the recommendations in the report (96 out of 106[193]), and in February 1993 with Nichol set up a task group led by Tim Chessells, a Regional Chairman, and Bob Nicholls, a regional manager seconded from Oxford, to take the changes forward. They formed the London Implementation Group (LIG), which co-ordinated the work of all four Thames regions with regard to health services in the capital. A series of specialty reviews was launched to sort out the 14 cardiac services, 13 cancer services, 13 renal services and the neuroscience services. Some would have to merge. For the next two years London was to take up a lot of headquarters time as ministers and officials fought their way through the professional and party politics. Along the way the London reforms redefined much of the planning context for the rest of the country.

The planning logic seemed impeccable. As patient length of stay reduced, efficiency improved and more and more surgery was undertaken in separate day-surgery centres, so the demand for traditional hospital beds would decline. At the same time the complex specialties needed to be centralised in order to conserve scarce skills and secure better clinical results. This process of centralisation also helped enormously in reducing the hours that junior doctors were expected to work. If you added to this increased investment in primary care, a new service could, it was generally agreed, be built with a very different shape. Other than the traditional hospital rivalries in London, the only fly in the ointment was an unexplained increase in medical emergencies and a marked reluctance by the public to sanction any concentration of Accident and Emergency services or agree any changes to their major hospitals. John Major was very exercised about London's health services. He could not understand why anybody would want to close or merge some of the country's leading hospitals. He gave Nichol a very hard time at a meeting with health ministers to discuss the matter by asking all the right questions. 'Don't give me the detail – tell me what the game is', he said to Nichol.[147] He was only half convinced by the answers, but as Nichol left the meeting in the Downing Street library, he put his arm around Nichol's shoulder and said 'You are doing OK.'

It was the plans for Bart's Hospital that attracted the most vigorous public argument. However, behind the scenes it was the merger of Guy's and St Thomas' Hospitals that was causing the trouble. Both were major national centres, but Guy's was in the ascendant professionally at this time. All of the London teaching hospitals knew that the only way to preserve their future was to acquire new populations to serve or pour concrete into new facilities, which would then have to be used. The London Implementation Group expected Guy's to be the main centre for the merged group. All of the big players were involved in the arguments, including the Prime Minister. Lord Harris, the Chairman of Guy's and his Chief Executive, Peter Griffiths (formerly the Deputy Chief Executive), were worried that their new high-tech block built primarily with money they had raised would in any merger be turned into an outpatient department. Lord Harris was a major fundraiser for the Conservative Party, so he was a voice to be listened to. St Thomas's had its own backers, including Virginia Bottomley, whose father had been Chairman of the Board. Duncan Nichol was a former deputy House Governor at St Thomas's. Ian McColl, a Guy's surgeon, was very close to John Major and would become his political secretary in the Lords. In the end the merger was forced through and Barney Heyhoe, the former Tory Minister, was appointed as Chairman. Bottomley and Nichol expected that Peter Griffiths would become the new Chief Executive, but this was not to be. The medical staff at St Thomas's doubted that they could work with him. (Griffiths went to the King's Fund and Tim Mathews from St Thomas's took over.) The principal tertiary specialties gradually moved to St Thomas's. They had won against the odds. These were political not managerial decisions.

The redevelopment of Guy's was later to cause substantial problems for the Executive when the PAC discovered that the costs had spiralled from £35.5 million in 1986 to £160 million in 1998.

The need to rationalise acute services in the major cities was not limited to London. Similar plans, based on much the same rationale as those for London, began to emerge in Birmingham, Manchester, Leeds and Newcastle. All of them involved building hospitals with fewer beds, centralising the inpatient component of many specialties and reducing the number of major Accident and Emergency centres. All of this caused much public disquiet, as the interested parties argued their case in public and the press took sides.

Search for focus

The search for focus is a recurrent theme of the Nichol years. In setting up the Management Executive, ministers had decided to try to limit themselves to long-term aims and directions, leaving specific objective setting and timing to local negotiation.[194] The new management arrangements were intended to focus both the Executive and health authorities on health outcomes and key priorities. The aim was to give regions the freedom to manage DHAs and FHSAs while enabling the Management Executive to hold regions to account for the achievement of objectives and services purchased for their populations. Nichol wanted a clear strategic plan for the NHS with agreed milestones against which progress could be judged.

In November 1990 the Policy Board had asked for a set of performance indicators that would enable it to judge the performance of the NHS. Six months later they adopted 15 indicators covering activity, manpower, finance and quality. The number was to be increased to 16 if purchasers were able to produce patient satisfaction data. The quality data were focused entirely on acute-sector waiting lists. Only the indicator about vaccination and immunisation targets for general practitioners had any connection to the core purpose of the NHS.

In August 1991, Nichol had demanded that all headquarter directors demonstrate that there was no disjunction between their day-to-day work and the Executive's strategic objectives.[179] The NHS performed well when given clear unambiguous targets. Waldegrave had asked for six or seven indicators of performance, and Roy Griffiths often spoke of the limited number he used to judge the performance of Sainsbury's. At this point many people seemed confident that the future management agenda would be dictated by the *Health of the Nation* strategy and the *Patient's Charter*.

This was, of course, far too idealistic. In practice it was a constant struggle. Every year it seemed that the guidance on what the centre wanted to see in short-term programmes grew. The management agenda was indeed enormous, as was the appetite of ministers for new initiatives and crisis response. The Treasury had made life complicated by insisting on the introduction of an efficiency index of performance in return for extra investment. Eventually it became perverse in its impact and put services such as community care and mental health at a disadvantage. The efficiency index became one of the most negative images of the reforms.

An extraordinary range of issues was dealt with by the NHS Management Executive at this time, both by the Executive itself and at the regular meetings they had with RGMs. Once the Executive had moved to Leeds, some meetings were held in London and some in Leeds. Between 21 July and 23 September 1992 the following four meetings show the wide range of topics considered.[195]

NHS Management Executive: minutes of 55th meeting on 21 July 1992

1 Performance pay
2 Capital distribution in the new NHS
3 Capital charges and weighted capitation
4 Technical change to the capital charge rules
5 Trust issues
6 Quality clinical management
7 GP prescribing
8 Consultant mobility

31st Policy Board meeting, 22 July 1992, Richmond House

1 Review of NHS general and senior managers' pay
2 London: Sir Bernard Tomlinson Inquiry

Joint meeting of Management Executive and RGMs, 10 September 1992

1 Corporate information report
2 Maternity services: response to the health committee report
3 Prescribing by GPs
4 NHS trusts fourth wave
5 Community care support framework
6 Information management and technology in acute hospitals
7 Supra-regional services
8 NHS breast screening services
9 National Blood Authority
10 RHA staffing
11 General and senior managers' reward package
12 Regional reviews
13 CMO group on specialist training

Secretary of State and regional chairmen's meeting, 23 September 1992

1 Quarterly performance report
2 GP prescribing
3 National Blood Authority
4 Community care
5 Other business: capital allocations, waiting lists, dentistry, black and ethnic minorities

Three months later, in October, the Management Executive was discussing an entirely new range of topics.

NHS Management Executive: minutes of 58th meeting on 27 October 1992

1 Health promotion and GP contract
2 Annual financial planning forum
3 Health of the Nation focus groups' reports
4 Development of Community Health Councils
5 Top-sliced budgets
6 Handling tertiary referrals: patients
7 Review of contracting
8 Regional reviews

Executive powers

Like its predecessors, Nichol's Executive took no decisions but provided advice to ministers and co-ordinated the day-to-day implementation of policy. It did, however, generate some space for itself and begin to shape policy in some areas, rather than just implement it. It was the Executive that decided to get to grips with the need for a National Information Strategy and put together the team that wrote it. At the end of the day it needed to be blessed by ministers, but that was all it was. It was Sheila Masters who made it plain that underlying deficits were simply not acceptable, and she enforced her view via the accountability review process. Left to follow their own instincts, ministers would have been more flexible and weighed the political consequences of zero tolerance. It was Nichol who encouraged innovation in the quality territory and found cash for national pilot schemes.

There was no formal statement of delegated powers, and there were no rules about authority or the powers of individuals. The rules that did exist related to the respective powers of the Department of Health and the Treasury. Nichol operated intuitively. Some problems had an obvious political dimension and went to ministers. Others he dealt with and, if appropriate, kept a minister informed about them. Many decisions were made and policy was created in the gaps and cracks of the formal processes. What did not help sometimes was the tradition whereby even junior civil servants reported directly to ministers in the areas in which they were working, often bypassing the Executive altogether.

Bottomley took the view that chief executives 'needed authority and stature in their own right, which meant they should be able to hire and fire, they should take credit when appropriate and have a certain degree of autonomy.'[167]

She claimed that she felt 'In many ways like an Executive Chairman with a chief executive who was a colleague rather than a side-kick.'[167] She would later veto any ideas about the NHS becoming an agency, but was happy to go a little way down the path of devolved authority. She even acknowledged that from time to time the Chief Executive might have to take a different view from her on a matter of policy, and that this might have to become public knowledge. In practice this was a very unlikely event, but the acknowledgement that it might happen is interesting after the events following the *Daily Mail* interview.

Bottomley took a similar view about the role of CMOs, whom she sometimes referred to as double agents. Their prime loyalty was to the integrity of their profession and the public health, and this in her view 'was a huge safety check on the authority, power and control of the Secretary of State.'[167]

Regions and the intermediate tier

In the spring of 1992 ministers and Nichol began to talk about the management structures that controlled and regulated the internal market, with a view to streamlining the organisation and reducing the management overhead. Concern about the language was also surfacing by May 1992. The term 'internal market' was being replaced by 'healthcare system.' As the number of trusts expanded it was becoming clear that the outposts which had been created to monitor them in January 1992 would be unable to cope. In any case a cross-over point at which purchasers and providers met, based at the centre, was too remote to work. The Trust Federation strongly resisted any ideas about a return to regional account-ability. They wanted no intermediate tier at all. Trusts were, they claimed, already sufficiently accountable to their boards, to purchasers, to the Secretary of State and to the public via their Annual General Meetings.

Ministers and the Management Executive discussed these issues in some detail at an away-day at Chevening in July 1992. They reached the following conclusions.

- There would be an intermediate tier.
- It would be statutory,
- It would be different from the Regions' light touch.
- It would be the cross-over point in the lines of purchaser management and provider regulation.
- It would create equal status for purchasers and providers.
- Market regulation would be designed to stimulate competition.

The idea of an independent corporation had been considered briefly, but Bottomley was not enthusiastic. All that would happen, she claimed, is that yet another body would be created to spend its time knocking on the Government's door for cash.

In July 1992 Nichol presented detailed proposals to the NHS Policy Board.[196] He spelt out clearly what the role of the new tier would be. Purchasers needed development and support but had to be held to account for securing, via contracts, national policy objectives and targets. Providers needed a lighter touch that was limited to ensuring they achieved their statutory duties (mainly financial) and conformed to the core values of the NHS. However, trusts did have to accept the realities of life, which meant that a 'political override' was ever present, even if it was rarely used. Market regulation should stimulate competition. In addition, the new tier would oversee the development of primary care. There was also a major debate about common services (estate, information, press and public relations, etc.) that were required by both the purchasers and providers, but no conclusions were reached.

Nichol also wanted to sort out the accountability confusion at the top of the NHS. The ambiguity in the position of RHA managers who reported both to the chief executive and to their own boards and chairman needed to be clarified. 'There must be,' Nichol argued, 'a direct and clear line of executive accountability down from the chief executive to the intermediate tier and to purchasing authorities and trusts.'[196]

The overlap of functions between the Department of Health and the regions also had to be tackled. This meant a parallel overhaul of the Management Executive. A review was commissioned led by Kate Jenkins, a member of the Policy Board, supported by Alan Langlands, the Deputy Chief Executive.[197] Jenkins had been head of the Prime Minister's Efficiency Unit from 1986 to 1989, when she left to become Personnel Director of the Royal Mail.

Nichol's paper was broadly accepted, but Bottomley continued to reflect on the recommendation to remove the regional tier. However, she did make some changes to the role of the Policy Board. She saw it as having two functions:

1 determining medium- and long-term policy in relation to the management of the NHS
2 setting objectives and reviewing their achievement by the Executive.

She did not want the Board to advise her on what to do about AIDS (she had others to advise her about this). She wanted the Board to focus on issues such as effective purchasing, the future of primary care, quality strategies, complaints, pay and communications. The Board was now focused very tightly on the NHS and its management, and from this point in time a representative from the Downing Street Policy Unit started to attend meetings on a regular basis.[198]

Stock-take

In February 1993 the NHS Executive met in Wetherby for one of the regular meetings with the regional general managers. Things seemed to be going well. The principles of the NHS had survived and overall investment was slowly increasing. The market had not imploded, the Patient's Charter had been launched successfully, and a new strategy for nursing was nearly ready. The trusts were beginning to perform, fundholding had started well, and the balance of power was beginning slowly to swing towards primary care. The *Health of the Nation*[138] had offered a coherent strategic framework for the purchaser arm of the system, and 100 additional consultant posts had been announced.

The capital programme was rolling on with over 100 schemes valued at over £1 million. Many of these schemes were funded in part or in whole from land sales. However, some schemes were proving troublesome, particularly those in London. One in particular, the new hospital in Kensington and Chelsea, attracted attention from the National Audit Office. It was the biggest contract ever let at £178 million, and it was overrunning badly.

There were still some problems with nurse grading appeals, securing jobs for newly qualified nurses and, most difficult of all, persuading the public to believe that things were actually getting better.

The structure of the NHS at this stage was as shown in Figure 4.3.

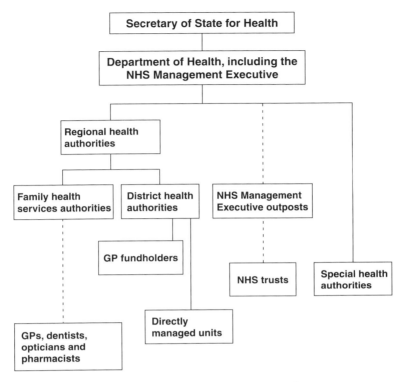

Figure 4.3 Structure of the NHS in England during the period 1991–96.

With the benefit of hindsight, Nichol is refreshingly straightforward about some of the early mistakes in presenting the reforms, saying that they spent too much time explaining what a market was rather than why it was necessary and what it might achieve.[147] They got the language wrong from the start. For the most part the public as well as the staff of the NHS associated the market with cost cutting and efficiency rather than with quality and responsiveness.

Support services

The early 1990s saw major changes in some of the major support services in the NHS. The expenditure by the NHS on external suppliers for goods and services was, at this time, around £4 billion annually, plus a further £2 billion on pharmaceutical products. The supplies function had been transformed and a network of new warehouse and distribution centres had been established to replace thousands of hospital stores. By 1993, NHS Supplies had reduced the number of hospital stores in England to 33 and had decreased the number of staff by around 1000, with consequent savings of around £27 million. The supplies service gained a professional edge as it drew into its ranks experienced people from the commercial sector. Information technology was exploding into the health sector and created real difficulties for NHS managers, who were by now trying to maximise the limited resources that they had for investment.

Reshaping the regions and the centre

In February 1993, the regions were told to reduce their staff to around 200 each by no later than 31 March 1994. For some this meant shedding hundreds of staff. The process of outsourcing whole divisions of regional staff to the private sector accelerated, including estates, management services, legal services and computing. Some did it badly, which led a year or two later to PAC appearances for Nichol and others who had been involved. Some regions began to look around for new and smaller headquarters. It was not the place to be in the NHS for young managers or professionals with careers to develop. Not everyone agreed with Nichol's conclusions. Roy Griffiths was not at all sure, for he understood the value of a buffer zone between ministers and the field authorities. Bottomley liked the idea of a local trouble-shooter (regional chairman) who believed with a passion in the Government's policies. However, the tide was turning strongly against the regions despite the continued close relationship between their chairmen and ministers.

The scandals in Wessex and the West Midlands had severely dented the Regions' reputations, and problems were beginning to emerge elsewhere, including London, where the boundaries of four regions met.

The detailed shape of the new intermediate tier was finally sorted out by Duncan Nichol and Brian Mawhinney, the Minister for Health, on a serviette in an Indian restaurant in Longsight, Manchester. They settled on eight organisations. Most fell into place naturally, but North London, East Anglia and Oxford were a problem. Mawhinney was a Cambridgeshire MP and did not favour any link with London. As a result, the new and very unwieldy Anglia and Oxford Region emerged.

By October 1993 the work of the Jenkins Functions and Manpower Review had been completed. Langlands recalls the process as being very hard fought and sometimes acrimonious. He was determined to get what he wanted and he largely succeeded. Twelve different working groups involving both civil servants and senior staff from the NHS had spent months working through the detail. The objective was to create within the Department as discrete an empire as was possible for the Executive. They wanted it to look and feel like the headquarters of the NHS. Bottomley made a statement in the Commons on 21 October 1993 in which she announced what she called the 'final stage of the reforms introduced in 1991.' The Plan was released to the staff under the banner *Managing the New NHS*.[140]

NHS: a new headquarters

Work began immediately on restructuring the NHS Management Executive to make it more clearly the headquarters of the NHS.

Fourteen regions were to be reduced to eight on 1 April 1994 and abolished altogether in 1996. The shell of the old regions would be maintained until 1996 to avoid primary legislation. The regional fiefdoms were to be replaced by a single corporate structure at the centre of the NHS with eight regional offices. A new power was sought that would enable district health authorities to merge with FHSAs. For the staff of regional offices it meant transfer from the NHS into the

Civil Service. No one was clear about what jobs would be available. Morale plummeted and good staff began to leave.[199]

Regional chairmen remained in the interim, but after 1996 they would stay on alongside the regional directors as what Bottomley called her 'Lord Lieutenants', who could 'act as the eyes and ears of the Secretary of State and tell her what she did not want to hear.'[167] This was despite the fact that their boards had disappeared. They also joined a revamped Policy Board. It was yet another fudge that never really worked, and the chairmen quite quickly took on a much more limited role as ministerial advisers on the selection of new members for the authorities and boards in their patch. The accountability chain between the Management Executive and the NHS remained opaque. Virginia Bottomley retained the ultimate responsibility to Parliament for the performance of the NHS.[140]

The Banks Review

While all of this was going on another review, of the wider Department of Health, was being conducted by Terri Banks, a former civil servant.

The Banks Review,[142] which was conducted at a time when Ken Clarke as Chancellor was demanding significant manpower reductions, divided the Department of Health into three business areas covering the NHS, Social Care and Public Health, each combining the responsibility for policy and implementation. At last within the NHS policy and implementation were to be merged. Those who developed policy had to pay regard to the difficulties and costs of implementation. The policy division, which had been at the core of the traditional Civil Service structures inside the Department, was to be broken up. For the Management Executive it offered the prospect of a distinct identity of its own within the Department, with a head who had direct access to ministers. Another huge internal reorganisation was about to occur.

At this point the Department of Health had 4690 staff, but substantial reductions were on the way as the Government concluded a wider review of Civil Service numbers. A 21% reduction was finally agreed in November 1994. The NHS Executive now had more civil servants working for it than the wider Department of Health, and the balance of senior appointments (at deputy secretary level) was weighted towards the Executive.[27] The principal casualty in all of this was the medical division. Integrated working meant a sharp reduction in the number of staff working directly to the CMO.[27] Donald Acheson, who had been CMO from 1983 to 1991, was later to allege in his evidence to the Bovine Spongiform Enchephalitis (BSE) Inquiry that 'his successors had been penalised and their independence compromised by staff cuts and restructuring in the DoH.'[200]

In the NHS some of the old arguments kept reappearing. The TV programme *World in Action* featured a survey in which one in three surgeons at the Alexandra Hospital, Redditch, said that they had been told to deal 'only or selectively with fundholders.'[201] In Birmingham the secretary of the local Medical Committee alleged that patients had to wait an additional five weeks for radiotherapy if they were not on a fundholder list. The market was still proving difficult to control, and there was also the problem of dealing with 'the laggards', as Nichol called them.

These were, on the one hand, purchasers who concentrated too much on organisational detail and too little on meeting the needs of their population, and on the other, providers who thought that they had a captive set of buyers. Nichol had by now concluded that 'the central dilemma was the reconciliation of the demand of parliamentary accountability and the delivered national policy, with the need to derive maximum benefits from the operation of the internal market.'[147]

By March 1994 Nichol had made up his mind to go. Major had offered him another term, but he declined on the grounds that he had done five hard years and had received a very good offer of a Chair in International Healthcare Management at the University of Manchester. He also knew an election was coming and that if Labour won, the reform programme would be quickly reversed. He wanted no part of that. Shortly after he had left a retirement party was organised at St Thomas's Hospital. All the Secretaries of State with whom he had worked attended and paid tribute to his skill. Ken Clarke was particularly warm in his appreciation.

Langlands was also generous in his praise of Nichol's leadership and drive in 'introducing the health reforms, probably the biggest challenge in the public or private sectors.'[202] Nichol had walked a difficult path in Whitehall, but under his leadership the NHS Executive had reformed the NHS in a way that few had thought possible at the outset. For this he had earned the respect of the politicians and managers with whom he had worked.

Chapter 5

Timeline

1994

March

- Alan Langlands took over as Chief Executive with Ken Jarrold as his Director of Personnel and his deputy.

April

- The new NHS Executive was created including regional directors as members.
- A total of 419 NHS trusts and 9000 GP fundholders were now in place.
- Eight regional health authorities doubled up as regional offices of the NHS Executive.

May

- The review of the wider Department of Health (Banks Report) published.[142]

August

- Virginia Bottomley stayed on as Secretary of State after a Cabinet reshuffle, with Gerald Malone as her Minister for Health.

October

- A major extension of fundholding and the concept of primary-care-led purchasing were announced as a major policy platform.
- *Managing the New NHS: a background document*[203] was published by the Department of Health.

November

- Sweeping staffing cuts of 21% were announced in the wider Department of Health.
- Regional offices, the old RHAs, were limited to a maximum of 200 people each.

December

- The Department of Health published the market rules, *The Operation of the NHS Internal Market: local freedoms, national responsibilities.*[204]

1995

January

- Doctors' and managers' leaders met in an attempt to re-establish effective working relationships.

February

- The King's Fund argued politically that the Government's plans to rationalise services in London were seriously flawed.

March

- Industrial action was threatened as some trusts refused to top up the national pay award of 1% to 3% without performance targets being first agreed. The Trust Federation reported confusion among its members over local pay, and called for a firmer national lead.

April

- The Calman–Hine Report (*A Policy Framework for Commissioning Cancer Services*)[205] was published by the Expert Advisory Group on Cancer to the Chief Medical Officers of England and Wales
- Bottomley announced plans for reshaping London's health services.
- London Conservative MPs revolted at plans to close St Bartholomew's Hospital and Guy's Accident and Emergency department.

June

- Shadow Health Secretary Margaret Becket ruled out the idea that Labour would support the Private Finance Initiative, dubbing it 'the thin end of the wedge of privatisation.'

July

- Stephen Dorrell took over as Secretary of State, with Gerald Malone as Minister of Health. Virginia Bottomley moved to become Secretary of State for National Heritage.
- Ken Jarrold encouraged trusts to bypass national pay negotiators and offer local pay deals.

August

- Ministers declared war on paperwork in general practice.
- Langlands told those health authorities that had made improper severance payments to seek to retrieve the money from the individuals concerned.

September

- Berkshire Health Authority was criticised for its plans to ration services because of a major review overspend.
- The Healthcare 2000 Report chaired by Sir Duncan Nichol (and funded by the pharmaceutical industry) agreed that rationing of health services was inevitable.[206]
- The Royal College of Physicians asked for a national body to advise on health service rationing.
- A deal was finally negotiated between the Department of Health and the trade unions that allowed local pay to be determined within a national framework.

October

- Harriet Harman took over as opposition spokesman on health.
- Stephen Dorrell demanded a further reduction in NHS management costs.
- Child B was denied treatment for leukaemia by Cambridgeshire Health Authority.

November

- Charles Webster published *The Health Services Since the War. Volume 2*.[207]

1996

January

- The Trust Federation called for a radical shake-up in the way that the internal market was organised. They wanted contracting simplified, access to capital made easier and lighter-touch monitoring of performance.

March

- Regional health authorities were abolished. The NHS Executive created eight regional offices.
- A number of trusts were reported to be in such significant difficulty that if they had been in the private sector the administrators would have been sent in.
- The Executive released a report on financial irregularities at Yorkshire RHA.[248]

April

- District health authorities and family health service authorities merged.
- A row about improper payments made to staff of the former Yorkshire RHA hit the national press.

July

- Labour announced plans to save £800 million from management costs as a first step in government should they be elected.
- The CBI complained about the red tape associated with the Private Finance Initiative.

August

- *Health of the Nation* was to incorporate the impact of the environment on health.
- Chris Smith became opposition spokesman on health and announced plans to return to national pay bargaining should Labour win the next election.

November

- Stephen Dorrell published *The National Health Service: a service with ambitions*,[208] which argued that the NHS was affordable.
- Dorrell reconstituted the Policy Board to accommodate regional chairmen.

December

- Dorrell announced an extra £25 million to cope with winter difficulties. The settlement for health authorities was 2% in real terms.

1997

January

- Financial deficits in trusts climbed to record levels.
- A total of 20 000 NHS managers were told that they could not have a pay rise.
- A snapshot survey showed that medical admissions were up 37% on the previous year.

March

- The NHS Confederation was created to represent health authorities and trusts. Philip Hunt was appointed as Director and Chief Executive of the Confederation.

May

- Ken Jarrold left his post as Director of Human Resources and Deputy Chief Executive and NHS Deputy, and became Chief Executive of Durham DHA.
- Labour won the General Election. Tony Blair became Prime Minister and Frank Dobson took over as Secretary of State, with Alan Milburn as Minister for Health and Tessa Jowell as Minister for Public Health.

July

- The NHS got a good three-year financial settlement (£21 billion).
- Frank Dobson demanded a purge of 'Tory deadbeats' from NHS Boards.
- Tessa Jowell announced an overhaul of *Health of the Nation*.
- A total of 15 new clinical indicators were added to the NHS performance league tables.

August

- Princess Diana died in Paris.
- National pay determination was confirmed, but not for staff on existing trust contracts.
- Philip Hunt left the NHS Confederation to become Labour Peer and Health Minister.

October

- Greg Dyke was brought in by the Government to advise on the updating of the Patient's Charter.

November

- There was growing public concern about failures and mistakes in screening programmes that were widely reported in the media.
- Waiting-list hit squads were appointed by the Department of Health.
- Graham Hart retired from the Civil Service and was replaced as Secretary of State by Christopher Kelly.

December

- Dobson launched the White Paper *The New NHS: modern, dependable,* with plans to abolish the internal market and create a new NHS based on primary care commissioning groups.[209]
- The report of the Committee of Inquiry into the Personality Disorder Unit at Ashworth Special Hospital (The Fallon Report)[210] was published.

1998

January

- Norwich Private Finance Initiative scheme (£214 million) was approved by ministers.

February

- Dobson announced that he had saved St Bartholomew's for the nation by refusing to agree to its closure.

March

- Milburn announced plans to change the Consultants Distinction Award system.
- *Our Healthier Nation*[211] was published.

April

- Ministers named the first 11 Health Action Zones.
- The trust merger trend accelerated.

June

- Sir Graham Hart became Chairman of the King's Fund in London.
- Ann Widdecombe became opposition spokesman on health, replacing John Maples.
- Bristol Royal Infirmary doctors involved in the paediatric cardiac surgery problem were struck off or disciplined by the General Medical Council.
- Milburn received a standing ovation at a conference of junior doctors in response to his promises to reduce working hours, improve access to part-time consultant posts and provide better food in hospital canteens.
- Stephen Thornton took over as Chief Executive of the NHS Confederation.

July

- The Chancellor announced an £18 billion increase in allocation for the NHS.
- The NHS celebrated its fiftieth anniversary in Westminster Abbey.
- Dobson launched a new quality initiative, *A First Class Service*.[212]

August

- Dobson announced a major reform of the Consultants Distinction Award system.
- Dobson authorised combined health and social service budgets.
- A £35 million expansion of NHS Direct was announced.
- New IT and human resource plans were launched.
- Dobson announced a public inquiry into children's heart surgery at Bristol Royal Infirmary.

October

- Dobson announced the Hospital Beds Inquiry at the Labour Party Conference.[213]
- Liam Donaldson took over from Sir Kenneth Calman as Chief Medical Officer.

November

- The Acheson Report, *Independent Inquiry into Inequalities in Health*, was published.[214]
- A league table of hospital costs was published.

- Dobson announced a £250 million uplift in NHS revenue allocations in order to enable the NHS to cope with winter pressures.

December

- Greg Dyke presented his report *The New NHS Charter: a different approach.*[366]

1999

January

- John Denham was appointed Health Minister, and Alan Milburn became Chief Secretary to the Treasury.
- The Department of Health issued guidelines limiting the prescription of Viagra.

March

- Langlands' contract was renewed for a further five years.
- The Royal Commission on Long-Term Care, chaired by Sir Stewart Sutherland, called for free personal care to be made available from general taxation.
- Blair called a meeting in Downing Street to discuss the sharp rises in outpatient waiting times.

April

- The National Institute for Clinical Excellence (NICE) started with Andrew Dillon as its first chief executive.
- A new minimum wage was announced.
- The Health Act replaced fundholding with primary care groups.

July

- Lord Philip Hunt, former Chief Executive of the NHS Confederation, was appointed to the ministerial team alongside Gisela Scott MP.
- *Saving Lives: our healthier nation*[285] was published.

August

- The Commission for Health Improvement (CHI), led by Pete Homa, began work.

October

- Alan Milburn was appointed as Secretary of State. The Public Health Minister post was downgraded and filled by Yvette Cooper MP.
- The National Institute for Clinical Excellence recommended that the flu drug Relenza should not be made available on the NHS.

December

- Neil McKay became Deputy Chief Executive of the NHS.
- NHS Direct took 113 500 calls during Christmas week.
- Milburn announced an inquiry into retained organs at Alder Hey Hospital.

2000

January

- The NHS survived the Millennium bug.
- Lord Winston created a storm about the treatment of his mother and inadequate levels of investment in the NHS.
- Tony Blair committed his Government to match European average spends on healthcare.
- GP Harold Shipman was found guilty of 15 murders.
- A total of 141 nurse consultant posts were created (a further 91 such posts were created in June).

February

- Alan Langlands announced his intention to resign and take up a new post as the Principal of Dundee University.
- The Beds Inquiry was published. Milburn responded with a pledge to open more hospital beds and create a new tier of intermediate care.[105]
- Primary care trusts struggled with escalating drugs expenditure that threatened to soak up all growth.

March

- Blair removed barriers to the NHS buying spare private-sector capacity. Milburn announced £600 million of additional money 'without strings' for England's NHS.
- Modernisation teams began to prepare the NHS Plan.
- Blair warned managers who could not or would not change that someone else would run the show.
- The Government announced plans to cut deaths from heart disease by 40% within 10 years.

April

- The Commission for Health Improvement produced a highly critical report on North Lakeland Healthcare Trust, the chairman of which was sacked.
- Milburn announced the membership of modernisation teams.

May

- Managers at Plymouth were suspended for under-reporting the number of patients waiting for more than 18 months.

July

- The NHS Plan[378] was launched.
- Doctors 'firmly rejected' the idea that newly qualified consultants should be barred from private practice for seven years.
- The Government responded to the Royal Commission on Long-Term Care.

August

- The Community Health Councils launched a campaign to block their abolition.
- Lord Hunt sent his 'hit teams' into seven trusts with long waiting lists.

October

- Nigel Crisp was appointed to the combined post of Chief Executive and Permanent Secretary.

November

- Milburn signed a concordat with private and voluntary healthcare providers.
- Neil McKay's post was upgraded to Director of Operations for the NHS.
- Colin Reeves retired as NHS Finance Director.

December

- Blair announced the winter plan for the NHS.
- The Health and Social Care Bill published *Putting Patients at the Heart of the NHS*.[379]
- The Conservatives promised to match Labour pound for pound in health and education investment.
- The White Paper *Reforming the Mental Health Act* was published.[380]

2001

January

- *Your Guide to the NHS*[215] replaced the Patient's Charter.

April

- An additional 1000 medical school places were announced, and two new medical schools.
- Milburn decided to wind up the NHS Executive and Regional Offices.

June

- The General Election kept Labour in power.
- Professor Paul Corrigan was appointed as political adviser to the Secretary of State. Simon Stevens, his predecessor, moved to Downing Street.

November

- The interim Wanless Report[325] was published, confirming that the NHS was the best economic model.

2002

January

- Milburn started to redefine the NHS with a speech to the New Health Network.
- The foundation hospital policy was launched.

March

- The Royal Commission on Long-Term Care reported.
- The Bristol Inquiry into deaths following paediatric cardiac surgery opened.
- *Delivering the NHS Plan: next steps*[334] was published.

April

- A historic funding decision was made to take investment to 9.4% of GDP by 2008.
- Primary care trusts took control of over 50% of NHS funding.

2003

February

- Milburn made a speech, *Localism: from rhetoric to reality*.[338]

April

- Four Regional Directors of Health and Social Care were appointed in line with *Shifting the Balance of Power in the NHS*[381] as the key functions of regional offices moved to the new strategic health authorities.

July

- Ian Bogle, the BMA leader, attacked the Government for providing 'care based on numbers and corporate bullying.'
- Alan Milburn resigned and John Reid took over as Secretary of State.
- A new Management Board was created at the Department of Health.

October

- Staffing cuts of 30% were announced for the Department of Health.

Alan Langlands, 1994–2000

Alan Langlands applied for the top job on the retirement of Duncan Nichol in 1994. He had been deputy for almost two years. Graham Hart, the Permanent Secretary, co-ordinated the process and joined the selection committee. The short list included Brian Edwards, by then Regional Director for the West Midlands, and Ken Jarrold from Wessex. Following a full suite of psychometric tests, the interviews took place in the office of Sir Robin Butler, the Head of the Civil Service, who acted as chairman. Sir Graham Day was present, as was the president of the Royal College of Physicians, but Roy Griffiths was again excluded. Langlands had worked hard as deputy and was a natural choice. As Joe Pilling, who was then the Principal Establishment Officer, expressed it:

> It seems to me, with the benefit of hindsight, clear that everybody else knew the plot but I did not. Crucially, Duncan Nichol and Graham Hart seemed to know the plot and Alan worked like nobody I have ever known in my career. At that point he was carrying a huge burden and was waiting to inherit his kingdom, which he eventually did.[91]

It was Langlands' name that duly went up to John Major for approval. There was the usual foul-up when Nick Timmins, the journalist, got hold of the result early and the announcement had to be rushed out. Langlands took over formally in March 1994.

Sir Alan Langlands, 1994–2000[216]

Alan Langlands was born in Glasgow in 1952 and educated in Allan Glen's School. He graduated in science from the University of Glasgow, and in 1974 he joined the national administrative training scheme with the NHS in Scotland. In 1981 he moved to London as Unit Administrator at the Middlesex Hospital, and became general manager of Harrow Health Authority in 1985. He was not enthused by the prospect of an internal market, and in 1989 he joined Towers Perrin as the leader of their healthcare consultancy arm. He acted as a consultant to the Northwest Thames Region in their preparations for change, and took over as RGM on the early retirement of David Kenny on health grounds in 1991.

In 1993, Duncan Nichol decided that he needed a deputy who could act as Chief Operating Officer and mop up the day-to-day issues while Nichol spent more time on the bigger strategic problems. Langlands was appointed to this new post on a secondment basis. He became Chief Executive in 1994 at the age of 43 years, and he received a knighthood in 1998. In 2000 he resigned to become the Vice-Chancellor of the University of Dundee.

Bottomley, the Secretary of State for Health, was not part of the selection panel, although she had undoubtedly been consulted about the short list. However, she did claim a power of veto. 'I was,' she claimed, 'entitled to know the process, satisfy myself on the process and, had there been a particular candidate that I felt it would have been impossible for me to work with, then to exercise a veto.'[167]

Langlands knew what the job entailed, and the handover from Nichol was straightforward. He understood from the start that his was not a classic chief executive role in the commercial mode. He was an administrator working to politicians:

> I have watched every Secretary of State during my career leaving office and saying health services management and day-to-day operations should be distant from politics. It doesn't work. As long as the NHS is squarely in the public sector someone in my position is going to need a finely tuned political antenna.[216]

The public perception had also changed to reflect more accurately the political realities. As David Walk wrote in *The Times*, 'The chief executive of the NHS has a job like running General Motors or the Red Army, which means managerially the job is impossible and perhaps should be classed as a political administrator.' He judged there to be an ineradicable difference in outlook, culture, timing and philosophy between politicians and managers, and Langlands was, he said, 'unavoidably stuck between the two. Responsible to a Tory Minister for a service that was philosophically socialist.'

Langlands set his stall out early at the National Association of Health Authorities and Trusts (NAHAT) conference in January 1994. He was, he said, 'resolutely confident about the future of the service and its people.' The changes at the top of the NHS were designed, he promised, to encourage purchasers and providers, not to impede them. 'The centre would,' he explained, 'concentrate on doing fewer things better and would resist the temptation to intervene in operational matters.' He went on to say 'The job of the NHS and the ME is about resolving a pattern of problems: the impact of science and technology, the economic environment, relationships with the professions and the implementation of Government policies. It was not,' he stressed, 'about tackling single great issues.'[202]

Bottomley had in fact given him four prime objectives:

- ensuring that the quality of patient services was central to the work of NHS management
- improving NHS performance in terms of efficiency and effectiveness
- successfully handling strategic change in London and other major cities
- streamlining the central management of the NHS.

Langlands moved quickly to build his new team. While the negotiations with the Treasury were taking place, he invited all those who were eligible to apply for the new regional director posts. The field of competition was regional general managers, outpost directors, grade two civil servants and Management Executive directors. The interviews for regional directors were held in March 1994 by a panel that included Langlands, Nichol, Hart (the Permanent Secretary) and the appropriate regional chairman. They were to be senior Civil Service appointments with some on Grade 2, which was a matter for some comment and concern within the ranks of the career civil servants, who saw their promotion prospects being sharply reduced by an influx of outsiders.

Ken Jarrold had been appointed to the post of Director of Personnel, and he also acted as Deputy 'in areas of general management responsibility.' He chaired Executive meetings when Langlands was unavailable. Alasdair Liddell, another former RGM, became Director of Planning. The role of deputy never really worked. As Jarrold said, 'It became clear within weeks of taking up the post that nobody could ever be Alan's deputy, because he did not work like that.'[218]

Langlands' first Executive Board met on 21 March 1994.[219] There were no grand announcements. The message to the outside world was one of continuity and an opportunity to build on the achievements of the past five years. It was a Board filled with people who had a background in the NHS.

Executive Board, 1994

Chief Executive	Alan Langlands
Deputy and Director of Personnel	Ken Jarrold
Director of Finance	Colin Reeves
Regional Director, Trent	Keith McLean
Regional Director, West Midlands	Brian Edwards
Regional Director, Northern and Yorkshire	Liam Donaldson
Regional Director, North Thames	Ron Kerr
Regional Director, South Thames	Chris Spry
Regional Director, Mersey and Northwest	Robert Tinston
Regional Director, South and West	Penny Humphries (Acting) and later Ian Carruthers (Acting)
Regional Director, Anglia and Oxford	Barbara Stocking
Director of Planning	Alasdair Liddell
Director of Corporate Affairs	John Shaw
Director of London Implementation	Bob Nicholls
Chief Nursing Officer	Yvonne Moores
Medical Director	Graham Winyard

In July 1993, when the Functions and Manpower Review had been approved, it was agreed with the Treasury that it would be helpful if a statement could be produced which set out clearly the roles and relationships of the various parts of the Department of Health. This was eventually produced in May 1995. Although it makes it clear that the Secretary of State is the one who sets the aims and objectives for the Department, it goes on to add:

> The Secretary of State does not normally become involved in the day-to-day management of the NHS, but is consulted by the chief executive of the NHS Executive on the handling of matters that give rise to public or parliamentary concern.[220]

This was heralded as a major move in policy, and is reflected in the role described for the chief executive: 'The chief executive is responsible for and directly accountable to the Secretary of State for the management and performance of the NHS in England.'[220]

In reality this was yet another presentational fudge. Health authorities and trusts remained accountable to the Secretary of State, not the chief executive, and ministers continued to be presented with a myriad decisions to be taken by the established Civil Service machine.

However, chief executives of NHS trusts, DHAs and FHSAs were designated as accounting officers, accountable to Parliament through the chief executive of the NHS. This designation had been rejected in 1985, but now reflected what Langlands believed to be the reality of a decentralised NHS operating from a headquarters in Whitehall.

Far from seeing this as another step in the process of devolution, some trust chairmen viewed it as Langlands trying to impose his authority on trusts by the back door. As John Spiers, the controversial former chairman from Brighton, put it, 'I constantly worry about trust chief executives being managed down the EL [executive letter] line from the centre. I think Alan Langlands is setting himself an impossible task if he is going to try to manage 500 trusts.' He added, rather sourly, 'Being chief executive of the NHS should not be a very large job. Political responsibility lies with ministers and purchasing authority with purchasers.'[221]

Although the big decisions about structure had been made, the detail was testing. The size of the new regional tier was particularly hard fought, with the Treasury, now led by Kenneth Clarke, taking a very tough line. They wanted no more than 30 people in these new offices. The Executive, which had tried to size the role properly, demanded 135. The negotiations got nowhere until Bottomley persuaded Langlands to threaten to resign with her if the Treasury would not budge. For a man who had only been in post a matter of weeks this was a tough decision, as he could not be absolutely sure that their bluff would not be called. In the event it worked, and a deal was struck behind the scenes. The following day at the formal meeting between the Department and the Treasury, Clarke let the argument run for 30 minutes or so and then turned to his officials and said 'That's it, I have heard enough – give them what they want.' He then turned his fire on Graham Hart and the wider Department in search of economies.[216] Langlands remembers the date well, for on the same day Mawhinney moved to the Department of Transport, much to the relief of everyone in the Department of Health. He had been a difficult minister.

Although the Executive is described as 'the top management team', its role was purely advisory. Although described as 'a single corporate body which is responsible for the central management of the NHS above the level of purchasers and providers', it had no powers of its own.

Here again we have an attempt to clothe an advisory body with the cloak of an authority that it did not possess. Langlands captures the reality in the following exchange:

> I remember once chairing a meeting of the Executive whilst Duncan Nichol was away. It went well, and after the meeting Mike Malone-Lee agreed that it had. The Executive had made nine clear decisions. But he then looked me straight in the eye and said 'You know of course that half of these things are not going to happen.' We went through them. Most did indeed require some subsequent negotiation with ministers, or some side conversation with the Treasury. I tracked these issues for about 15 months, and I reckon we only got three

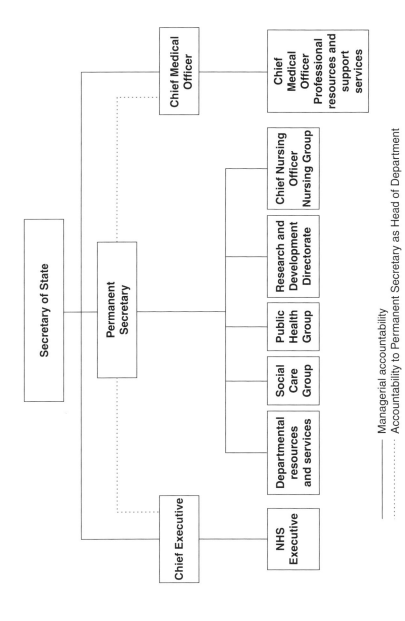

Figure 5.1 Structure of the Department of Health in 1995.[220]

and a half out of nine. The rest were either overturned by ministers or we went off in a different direction. Three and a half was a good batting average.[216]

Often the Chief Executive was not looking to his Board for decisions but for a sense of direction, a sounding board, support and sometimes comfort. The ability to argue that a particular course of action had strong board backing was sometimes helpful and influential with ministers.

However, regional directors had a job description that was unusually explicit. They were directly responsible for the performance of the health authorities in their region, and for monitoring the activities of trusts. The outposts were swept into the new regional offices, although some outposts held on to an independent line for some months and eventually had to be told by Langlands to identify themselves with the new organisation. Although regional directors were 'responsible', the chief executives of health authorities remained primarily accountable to their boards and their chairmen to the Secretary of State.

Langlands' style at these meetings was interesting. Sometimes he declined the chair and listened to the discussions. His name appears in the alphabetical list of those present, but does not identify him as being in the chair. He did not attend all of the meetings, and Ken Jarrold often found himself in the chair. Langlands tried very hard both to be an excellent civil servant and to maintain his credibility with NHS management. He identified himself as being the subject of Rudolf Klein's comment that 'no one is ever clear about whether he is the NHS's person in the corridors of power or the minister's person in the operating theatre.'[216]

In an unusual move he asked all the members of his team to go through a process of personality profiling so that everyone's strengths and weaknesses could be identified. For his early meetings and away-days he used an external facilitator.

He reported to the Board in December 1994 on a range of interviews that he had conducted with each Board member. Overall the conclusion was that the Board meetings and relationships were improving. However, there was some disagreement about what issues should be discussed by the Board. Most were interested in more focus on the forward agenda and future key priorities. Interestingly, regional directors were more positive about the role and purpose of the Board than directors based at headquarters.[222]

Another internal restructuring began in earnest. The precise role of the new regional directors had to be sorted out and their staffing structures graded and approved. The RHAs had to be formally closed down and decisions taken about which staff would be transferred to the new regional offices and which would have to go on redundancy or early retirement terms. The site of their offices had to be reviewed, and most made a physical change to smaller premises. The staff that transferred, including the directors, had to be assimilated into the Civil Service. There were to be no secondments this time. Inside the headquarters, changes and reductions were in progress. There was a determined attempt to make the new Executive a real headquarters for the NHS with a distinctive identity of its own within the Department of Health.[218] Some of those at risk had made the move from London to Leeds only a few years earlier. The headquarters of the NHS was to be a Civil Service organisation in its totality. Langlands moved his family to Yorkshire, but the rest of the directors stayed in London or elsewhere and commuted. This worked for a while, but eventually became very dysfunctional as Langlands and his team were almost constantly in London.

In December 1994, Langlands and his team published a definitive guide to the operation of the internal market.[204] It covered rules relating to mergers and joint ventures as well as the action that would be taken when providers got into difficulties. More controversially, it also dealt with what action would be taken to prevent inappropriate collusive behaviour by trusts. The market at last had some hard rules.

While all of this was happening, the Bill that became the Health Authorities Act 1995 was working its way through the parliamentary process. The Act abolished district health authorities and family health authorities with effect from 1 April 1996, and replaced them with new health authorities with responsibilities across the whole range of health services.

By this stage the quarterly monitoring of the NHS had increased sharply, and large volumes of data started to move up the system. The Department of Health now knew more about the day-to-day operations of the NHS than it had ever done before. What had started with activity and expenditure trends now incorporated prescribing trends, Patient's Charter adherence and waiting lists. The monitoring reports were classified as highly confidential.

A snapshot of NHS Executive business in 1994 is set out overleaf.

This was not a Board to handle the day-to-day business of the NHS. It met once or twice a month, often on a two-day basis. It had a long forward agenda that shaped up issues before they reached ministers. Langlands used it to communicate messages from ministers and to seek colleagues' views. Even on a complex issue such as weighted capitation (the formulae that decided revenue allocations to health authorities) there was a regular flow of traffic to ministers as the policy was developed. They were still very much in charge and made a number of changes to the recommended formulae. The most crucial change was to give a zero rating to the 24% of the budget that covered community and administrative services.[223] The capitation issue was important for two reasons. It signalled the final stage of regional power (until this point the Department had issued revenue to RHAs who then decided the apportionment among health authorities within their region) and it was a powerful centralising issue.

Handling revenue allocations nationally certainly added to the sum of ministerial power, but it carried its own dangers. When the new formulae were finally agreed, some columnists claimed that the principal beneficiaries were ministers' constituencies. The formulae certainly benefited the Home Counties and took some of the pressure off London. The Health Select Committee considered the formulae to be deeply flawed for this reason.

The Langlands Executive had no more formal powers than the Nichol Executive had had, although Langlands himself had clearer authority over his headquarters budget. He certainly influenced the resource allocations to the NHS, but he had no direct powers to intervene in local spending. In practice, he and Colin Reeves, his Finance Director, between them could usually find the money from some budget or other to do the things that they considered to be important. In this manner they seeded many initiatives in the NHS itself.

However, cash for the NHS was a perpetual problem throughout Langlands' term of office, despite the fact that the financial management of the NHS had, in just a few years, been transformed.

Snapshot of NHS Executive business in 1994

Business	21/3	25/4	5/5	23/5	2/6	20/6	7/7	18/7	1/9	19/9
Confidentiality	*					*				
Public Expenditure Survey	*									*
Weighted capitation	*	*	*	*					*	*
Planning guidance	*	*								
Mental health	*						*			*
Restructuring	*	*	*	*						
UK Central Council for Nursing		*								
NHS data flows		*			*					
Patient's Charter		*								
Waiting lists		*			*					
Specialist services			*					*		
League tables			*		*					
St Bartholomew's Accident and Emergency department			*							
Communications			*					*	*	*
Organisational development			*							
NHS Estates				*						
Cancer services				*		*				
Research and development				*		*				
Quarterly returns				*					*	*
Pay				*				*		*
Nursing at HQ				*						
Community Health Councils				*						
Health of the Nation					*					
European Community procurement					*					
Ethnic health						*				
Fundholding						*				
Prescribing						*				
Outpatients department standards						*				
Dentistry							*			
Quality							*			
Efficiency							*			
Coronary arterial bypass grafts							*			
Audit Commission							*			
Private Finance Initiative							*			
Handling parliamentary questions								*		
DHA/FHSA mergers								*		
Measles								*		
Relations with doctors								*		
Purchasing								*		*

The growth that had been injected into the NHS in the early years of the market had slowed sharply.

Langlands and Reeves kept a running graph showing the relationship between increased activity and new money. They understood that the consequences of years of low investment would come home to roost at some stage. Despite a huge increase in demand, the NHS bumped along with real growth rates of around 1%. GDP levels of investment in health were stuck at around 5.8%, far below those in most of the other countries in Europe.[224] Bottomley and Langlands fought hard for higher growth, but without much success. In 1995–96 it was 1.5%, and the following year it was 0.6%, which was well below the amount needed by the NHS to keep the books straight.

A report by C4 Consulting in March 1996 indicated that one-third of trusts were worth less than when they had been set up, and 14 trusts would have had the administrators sent in if they had not been in the public sector.[225] Only one trust went bust. This was Anglia Harbours, when it lost its principal contract.

However, ministers preferred to tell the simpler story about cash balancing across the system. 'End-of-year cash crises are part of the history of the NHS, not its future,' Bottomley claimed.[167] She was wrong. Only a little over a year later her successor was to inject extra cash mid-year in order to cope with a winter crisis.

In accordance with the Thatcher principles, Bottomley had kept her foot firmly on the efficiency accelerator. In 1995–96 she had demanded a 3% efficiency gain which, if achieved, would contribute £600 million to the development kitty. Some (perhaps most) of this gain was real, but much of it was non-recurrent and it was very difficult to confirm after the event what the real recurrent gain had been. However, the number did go into the Treasury as if it had been achieved, and was added to the £1.9 billion provided by the Treasury in any public announcements about NHS funding.

Local pay bargaining

The development of local pay structures had been a mainstream policy objective since *Working for Patients*[94] was published. John Major, the Prime Minister, had told Virginia Bottomley that there were two principal objectives which she had to deliver, namely the Private Finance Initiative (PFI) and local pay.[218] It was one of the most important trust freedoms, but progress had been slow. In June 1994, Langlands had told trusts to have local pay machinery in place by February 1995. By October 1994, 30% still did not have acceptable plans in place.[226]

The BMA urged its members to have nothing to do with local pay deals, and UNISON and the Royal College of Nursing had also signalled their disagreement. The Management Executive and the Policy Board discussed the issues involved in some detail in July 1994. Trust enthusiasm for local pay had cooled, they were told. Less than 20% of trust staff were on local pay. Many thought that the present position was ideal. There was a national agreement, but with flexibility to go local when it was useful to do so. Many managers worried about the potential for many local disputes and the creation of unfortunate precedents and a consequential pay spiral. The Executive decided to advise the Policy Board not to move against the Whitley system, and to spend more time explaining the benefits of local pay.

The row rumbled on, and in October 1994 UNISON offered a compromise of a national pay spine for trusts to adapt locally. It was not accepted. The policy commitment to local pay and PFI had to be delivered. Many within the Department and the NHS had doubts about the wisdom of pushing on. The intellectual arguments for moving down this road were robust. The doubts were whether local pay bargaining could be made to work with national pay bargaining and a powerful independent review body system still in place. Early in 1995, the review bodies of the nurses and the professions allied to medicine recommended a 1% pay rise to be topped up with local agreements valued at between 0.5% and 2%. These became known as X and y agreements (X being the national and y the local agreements). The unions wanted a further 2% with no strings attached.

The Trust Federation was undecided about its next steps. It reported uncertainty and confusion among its members. There were now doubts being expressed as to whether local pay was possible anyway without national enabling agreements. It all 'seemed to be moving too quickly,' said the Chairman of the Federation's human resource committee. 'Local and regional markets may well be an emerging trend, but we are not at that stage yet.'[227] Ideas began to circulate about local employer confederations and pay clubs. In April the Royal College of Nursing suggested that it might accept local pay if enough trusts (more than 300) offered a no-strings-attached 3% this time around.[228] UNISON remained opposed, and with others began to contemplate industrial action in September. Relationships between the RCN and the group of unions led by UNISON had by this stage become very strained indeed, which added a further complication to the negotiations.

By the end of June 1995, 429 of the 485 trusts employing nursing staff had made an offer, the majority (359 trusts) at 3%.[229]

Jarrold toured the country in July trying to persuade trusts to play ball and make local deals.[230] If the opportunity presented itself he would also talk to the media, even though this meant promoting a controversial policy about which he had his own doubts. He regarded it as part of his job to explain how the policy was designed to be in the interests of staff and patients. In retrospect he thought that he might have gone too far, but no one said as much at the time.[218] It helped a little when he was able to confirm that some new money would be available to meet the cost of local deals and it would not all have to come from efficiency savings. Most trusts wanted to include performance results in any local deal. Some trusts wanted strings,[231] while others would settle for threads. They included consolidating extra statutory holidays into annual leave, achieving targeted reductions in absenteeism and sickness, and meeting or maintaining Patient Charter standards. The unions simply wanted the extra 2% without strings.

Bob Abberley, the UNISON leader, told the National Association of Health Authorities that they should get involved, but they seemed reluctant to tread on the toes of the Federation. Philip Hunt, the Chief Executive, limited himself to arguing for a small x and a big Y, with the latter being the local component. As the summer progressed the trusts began to settle, although occasionally local staff sides had to withdraw from agreements that had already been made because of instructions from their national leaders. As the national pressure grew, many trusts agreed to make interim deals pending the outcome of national negotiations.

Eventually a deal was struck after 16 hours of talks in September 1995. This hinged on local pay within a national framework and a safety net, which in the view of the unions would limit local pay variations to a fraction of 1%. It was hailed by both sides as a victory for the NHS, but the unions were not really satisfied and the RCN was incensed at what it considered to be a stitch-up between UNISON and the Executive. The Trust Federation bemoaned their loss of autonomy. It would have been different, some claimed, if they had handled the negotiations rather than the Management Executive and ministers. Both sides went away to sell the deal to their constituencies, but it was a foregone conclusion. A deal had been struck that got both sides off an uncomfortable hook. In any case it was only a face-saver, because Chris Smith for the Labour opposition was already committing his party to a return to national pay bargaining if they won the next election.

The arguments started about the following year's pay process. Jarrold confirmed that he would recommend a national pay rise, while the Federation demanded a weakening of the national structures to give local pay a chance to develop.

Bob Abberley captured what he thought was the essence of the argument in an address to the NAHAT Conference in the same year (1996). Local pay means that you got 1970s British Leyland-style unions fighting for the best deal. 'It's a novel industrial relations concept,' he said when a trust chief executive told him, a union official, to go and see his purchaser who had all the money. 'It's like asking your opponent to do your job by appealing to the customer.'[232]

'We have,' Abberley told the delegates, 'ended up with the worst of all worlds. Demoralised, furious and mutinous staff, highly charged relationships between purchasers and providers, and a government that is now sitting back and washing its hands of the problems. It's a shambles.'[232]

Most managers agreed with him.

Other than occasionally offering advice the Executive had hardly been involved, except through Ken Jarrold, the Director of Personnel. He shuttled between ministers and the Trust Federation and the Chairmen of the Whitley Councils trying to establish a clear management line. Ministers were actively involved at every stage and they made all of the key decisions.

In October, Jarrold reported to the Policy Board that the problem had been largely resolved. The large unions had settled and 60% of trusts had already made interim payments. Now was the time, he argued, to encourage trusts to increase their investment in personnel management and be more enthusiastic about local bargaining.[233]

Jarrold, in a thoughtful retrospective, wishes that he had expressed his doubts about implementation more strongly than he did to ministers.[218] However, if he had done so he would have risked being branded as negative and his credibility within the Department being damaged. Ministers should have realised that local pay meant an end to most national negotiation and the demise of the Independent Review bodies. They declined the battle that was needed to bring this about, and the policy failed. Some trusts that had gone out on a limb to introduce local pay structures felt they had been sold down the river, while others blamed themselves. Roy Tyndall, the Human Resource Director at the Royal Liverpool

Hospital, told his colleagues 'the whole deal has been cobbled together because most trusts have failed to introduce local pay despite the opportunities they have had. First-wave trusts have had four years to get new recruits on to local contracts, and many have failed to act.'[234] He was right, but this had been plain for some time. Christine Hancock, the General Secretary of the RCN and herself a former manager, saw managers as victims of a pay dispute characterised from the start by government misinformation and mismanagement.[235]

This was a good example of an attempt to introduce a controversial policy without sensible anticipation of the nature and scale of the opposition.

Extensions to fundholding

One of the most challenging policy areas was GP fundholding, and by October 1994 ministers and the Executive were looking for a coherent development path once they had already decided in principle to go for a primary-care-led NHS. By this stage 41% of the population was covered and fundholding was judged by ministers to be one of the great success stories of the new NHS.[236] They decided to lower the list-size threshold for entry to 5000 and introduce a junior version for those with list sizes of 3000 or more who only wanted to purchase community services. They also launched 51 'total fundholding' pilot schemes in which GPs from a number of practices came together to purchase all hospital and community services for their patients. In taking these decisions, ministers in particular had been anxious to preserve a significant role for the new health authorities, which would come into being on 1 April 1996. Their role would include responsibility for implementing national strategy, answering the health needs of local populations, and monitoring GPs in their commissioning and providing roles. It was the health authorities that would police the new accountability framework for GP fundholding.

Challenges about two-tierism were never far away and seemed to put ministers constantly on the defensive; others argued along more robust lines. The Association of Fundholding Practices said 'Let it be clear, fundholders have created a two-tier service. They have shown what a top tier can do.'[225]

Allegations of Stalinist approach

Early in 1995, Langlands gave a series of interviews to the professional press. He had to respond to a growing series of reports that the Executive was remote and out of touch with the real world. An article in the *British Medical Journal* by Craft and others[237] alleged that the NHS was becoming Stalinist and that freedom of speech was being suppressed and consultants' telephones were being tapped. Langlands reacted strongly in a letter to the *British Medical Journal*, expressing his horror that there remained in the NHS people who felt they worked in a climate which prevented them from freely expressing their views.[237] That was not the sort of organisation he wanted to lead. His riposte was blunted somewhat a few days later by a survey in the *Health Services Journal* which found that more than 50% of managers believed that the NHS had become more secretive over the last five years. A large majority reported that their trust employment contracts had confidentiality clauses.[238]

The truth was uncomfortable. There was a strong sense, at least among managers and chairmen, of having to be on side in any dealings with the media. Chairmen in particular, having taken the Queen's shilling, had to support the cause or resign. Trusts kept their business plans very close to their chest and dealt with much of their business as 'commercial in confidence'. It was an inevitable consequence of the competitive environment in which they operated.

Langlands did spend a good deal of his time out in the field with NHS staff, and although this helped him to keep his instincts close to the real world, it did little for his national image. He was largely unknown to the general public. He was not a man for flashy initiatives or inspirational speeches; he valued clarity and coherence more.[239] He was not a man with a political passion for the market, but he did understand and value its power. 'This is not a game of winners and losers. It is about providing an important public service and using the dynamic of the market and the process of competition to stimulate improved efficiency.'[239]

Decisions about London

In April 1995, Bottomley announced her decisions about London. St Bartholomew's Hospital was to close as an acute site, along with the London Chest Hospital and the Brook Hospital. Greenwich Hospital and Edgeware General were to be run down and the Accident and Emergency department at Guy's Hospital closed. A total of £238 million was to be spent rebuilding and refurbishing the London Hospital at Whitechapel, and primary care was to be upgraded. There was an inevitable row, including a threatened revolt by six Tory MPs. Labour demanded a moratorium on all bed closures in the capital. The local Community Health Councils were deeply sceptical.[240] The plans were, they claimed, full of flaws and risks. However, primary care got a support team with £1 million a year cash for investment. The row about the future of St Bartholomew's continued. Wreaths were placed on the tombs of Rahere, the Augustinian monk and founder of Bart's. Taxis drivers were issued with 'Save Bart's' stickers, and Labour got in on the act when Margaret Beckett, then opposition health spokesman, toured the hospital's Accident and Emergency unit before it closed.

Smothering the market

By 1995, Bottomley had moved the NHS quite a long way from the internal market envisaged by Clarke and Thatcher. 'The NHS is not a business,' she told the Royal Society of Medicine in June 1995, 'the only profit it makes is measured in the cure of illness, the care of the sick, the relief of pain and its contribution to a healthy nation. We are all its shareholders; but our interest is human, not financial.'[362]

She went to considerable trouble to rebut a suggestion by Peter Griffiths that eventually all trusts should become fully independent not-for-profit organisations. However, as Nichol Timmins points out, when it came to community care she was insisting that 85% of the care element of earmarked cash given by central government to local authorities had to be spent in the independent sector.[111]

She was clearly drawing a line under 'the reforms' and building a new platform for change. The market had been effectively smothered.

Rationing and Child B

The debate about rationing in the NHS was given a major boost in September 1995 when a pharmaceutical industry-funded think tank chaired by Sir Duncan Nichol reported that rationing was inevitable in the NHS and should be done properly.[206] The Royal College of Physicians demanded a national rationing debate. Some health authorities began to define with considerable precision what they would fund and what they would not. Berkshire, an authority that was in deep financial difficulties, announced a blanket ban on inappropriate procedures.[241] A decision to decline to pay for the removal of tattoos caused little comment (although one Director of Public Health did argue that there could be overwhelming humanitarian reasons for doing this), but what about fertility treatment? The test of only paying for treatment that worked stumbled against the fact that much clinical practice was not underpinned by properly researched evidence. On the other hand, new drugs were an easier target to block until evidence became available that they worked and could be justified on economic grounds. In the West Midlands Region, a central committee chaired by a leading GP reviewed all new drugs, and some old ones, and made recommendations to the GPs in the region. One reason for doing this was to help those GPs who wanted to stop prescribing inappropriate drugs to insistent patients. At the centre these local decisions began to create problems as the opposition began to attack what it called 'postcode prescribing', whereby if a person lived on one side of the street the NHS would pay for their treatment, but if they lived on the other side they would not. The tension between local priorities and a national service was increasing with a vengeance. Ministers were becoming uneasy with aggressive purchasing. The Executive rejected any notion of a national list of proscribed treatments. Stephen Dorrell confirmed this line in his Millennium Lecture in Manchester. He did want the NHS to stop giving ineffective and unnecessary treatment, but there could be no blanket bans: 'There should be no clinically effective treatment which an HA decided as a matter of principle should not be provided. There would always be the exceptional case where treatment was clinically justified.'[242]

It was a young child from Sawbridge near Hertford who brought the issue to the forefront of national consciousness. To begin with she was identified as Child B, but later identified herself as Jaymee Bowen, aged 11 years, in a television interview for the *Panorama* programme. She had been diagnosed as having leukaemia and she underwent treatment, which was initially successful. However, three years later the cancer returned in a more virulent form. A bone-marrow transplant produced some immediate relief, but the effects did not last. The child became very ill. The specialists in Cambridge who were treating her thought that she had only weeks to live and judged the chance of a second bone-marrow transplant being successful to be 2% at best.[243] A second opinion from specialists in London confirmed this view. Jaymee's distraught father declined these judgements and found yet another specialist who was willing to try a new and experimental technique (donor lymphocyte infusion). Cambridgeshire

Health Authority refused to authorise payment for further treatment on the grounds that they had been advised that another attempt was not in the patient's best interests. It was not, in their judgement, an investment that they could justify, given the very small chance of success, and the other claims on their limited resources. The case ended up in the High Court, which ruled that the health authority should pay. This decision was almost immediately overruled by the Court of Appeal, which accepted the argument that in the hard world of the NHS, treatments which did not have much chance of success could not be realistically funded by the NHS. A large private donation ensured that Jaymee received the experimental treatment at a private hospital in London. Initially it was successful, and Cambridgeshire Health Authority agreed to fund Jaymee's continuing care, but she died the following year.

Panorama had interviewed Stephen Thornton, the Chief Executive of Cambridgeshire Health Authority, in October 1995. According to *The Sunday Times*, he came across as 'not uncaring but actuarial.' Jaymee's interview stole the show and evoked huge public sympathy. Asked what she would say if she met Stephen Thornton, her reply was unhesitating. 'I wouldn't sit there and say to him,' she retorted, 'I'd just go over there and whack him one.'[244] The leader in the *The Times* the following day was both supportive and challenging. It was accepted that although health authorities with finite resources were properly reluctant to spend money on unproven procedures, this represented a real problem for the future of medicine:

> The danger of orderly rationing is that no gambles will be taken, no hunches pursued. Every medical procedure that we now take for granted, from hip replacement to bypass surgery, was experimental at one stage. Nobody expects health managers to waste money on moonshine. Equally they must leave space for uncertainty and risk taking.[245]

However, Thornton did receive some credit for subjecting himself to 'a cross-examination of a kind which bureaucrats have rarely faced in the past.'

A few months later the Executive reviewed the case with Thornton and his team.[376] By now it was too late to influence events in any way, but the situation would no doubt occur again as these issues were becoming 'the warp and the weft of the health service.'[245]

Opinion was mixed. Some thought that Thornton and his authority had taken a brave stand on an issue of principle, while others thought that he should have quietly paid up, with an added requirement for an independent evaluation of the results. Yet others argued that once managers and politicians got this close to tough ethical decisions affecting individual patients, they almost always lost the argument. Managers and authorities ran the system and should not intrude at the level of the individual patient. On balance, the Cambridge case helped the moves towards evidence-based medicine and demonstrated in a very vivid manner that money was finite and modern medicine still did not have all the answers. The early thinking about a future National Institute for Clinical Excellence (NICE) began here.

The issue of rationing was one in which Langlands took a close personal interest. In the NHS annual report for 1994–95 he acknowledged that setting priorities was a fact of life: 'There will always be a gap between what the NHS might wish to do and that which is possible.' In what many saw as a move to distance himself from Nichol's report on the future,[206] he confirmed his view that 'the way forward was a tax-based service largely free at the point of delivery. That's the remit I am running with, and I believe I am going to be running with it for quite a long time.' He went further by adding the phrase that caught the headlines: 'I do distance myself, not just emotionally but logically from the ration-and-privatise brigade.'[246]

Langlands' conclusion was that if one had a robust framework for decision making one could begin to address some of these tough judgements about individual patients.

Community care

Community care was another area in which pressure had been growing for national definitions of patient entitlement. The numbers were startling. Over one million people were expected to live beyond the age of 85 years at the turn of the century.[208] This was a particularly sensitive area, as those who were judged to fall outside the criteria would have to pay for themselves if they had the resources. Many families saw their parents' assets being poured into expensive long-term care in nursing homes. By 1995 the NHS had sharply reduced its own continuing care capacity. Ministers had been reluctant to issue national criteria for eligibility, arguing that this was a matter best settled by health and local authorities, even though this would lead to patients with the same needs having their nursing-home bed funded by one authority but not by another. Critics argued that national criteria were the only way to maintain the founding principle of equity of access to NHS services. Variation between local authorities might be acceptable, but not in the NHS.[247]

Ministers stuck to their guns, but collaboration between the NHS Executive and the Social Services Inspectorate ensured that there was in practice a high degree of national consistency in the application of the criteria. Dorrell wanted to encourage a private insurance market in this field.

Tony Blair upped the political temperature at the Labour Party Conference in 1996 when he condemned a country in which the elderly had to give up their homes in order to acquire the care that they needed.[111] It was a statement that would influence the spending plans of his government when he came to power.

Sleaze again

Behind the scenes a problem had been developing involving Keith McLean, one of the regional directors on Langlands' new team. Prior to his appointment he had been Chief Executive of the Yorkshire RHA, which the District Auditor claimed had made irregular payments of relocation expenses to senior staff amounting to just under £0.5 million, and had incurred excessive hospitality expenditure. There was also criticism of a land sale, the letting of consultancy contracts and the provision of official cars. Langlands had set up his own inquiry, in the spring of 1995, chaired by Colin Reeves, his Director of Finance. This reported back to him in the autumn that McLean had 'failed to discharge his duty of care to the RHA and behaved in a manner unacceptable in a public servant.'[248] The report was made public in March 1996 by the National Audit Office, which had also shown a keen interest in the affair, not least because McLean's predecessor in Yorkshire, Andrew Foster, was by now the Comptroller of the Audit Commission.[249]

'Sleaze was back,' said the *Health Service Journal*, and its stain ran embarrassingly close to the upper echelons of NHS management.[248] McLean defended himself vigorously, although he had little time to construct his defence. He challenged the accuracy of the report. He had acted, he said, 'in the interests of the NHS' and although 'with hindsight some of his judgements may not have been correct, in other matters he would take the same decision.' McLean admitted that he 'embraced the culture of the day too enthusiastically and uncritically in pursuit of successful outcomes.'[250] But he also argued that others had done the same and 'the Department had actually pushed a general message to relax the rules in order to get things done.' It was a 'can do' culture and not a 'collective hallucination'. 'We are now in danger,' he said, 'of having the system administered rather than managed. There is a danger we will get unimaginative, cautious, non-inspirational management.'[250]

McLean could not stay on as a Director, particularly as it was already clear that a PAC hearing was inevitable. Langlands told the *Health Services Journal* that 'McLean has gone – not because he wants to avoid accountability but because I decided he was not a fit person to be an Executive Director in the new NHS.'[249]

Many in the NHS thought this to be a harsh judgement, as McLean did indeed have a reputation for getting things done. His career in the NHS was effectively over. Some judged that the penalty did not fit the crime. Langlands probably had little choice but to take the action he did. Given recent history he could not afford to allow even a breath of scandal to taint the Executive. The entrepreneurial spirit of the internal market had to be reined in, and people needed to be reminded that they were working in the public sector, which had sterner rules and standards.

Health of the Nation

The *Health of the Nation* policy[138] launched in 1992 was still active under Langlands and Calman, the new CMO. Although it was not easy to demonstrate a clear relationship between cause and effect (except perhaps for smoking cessation), by 1996 results were available to demonstrate some progress.[251] The Department of Health thought that this represented good progress but the National Audit Office was not very impressed, pointing out that 'good' progress had been made on less than half of the targets.[225]

The *Health of the Nation* targets continued to appear in the annual priorities and planning guidance, but by this stage the early passion had dissipated and the shorter-term agenda dominated the day-to-day life of NHS managers. However, evidence-based medicine was very much in vogue, and the Cochrane Centre and the NHS Reviews Centre were being accessed regularly by both clinicians and managers. Sometimes the results of the application of this new thinking proved controversial. Wiltshire Health Authority asked obstetricians to reduce the number of Caesarean births on the grounds of both safety and cost-effectiveness. There might be a slightly enhanced risk with a Caesarean birth, but it cost five times as much as a normal birth. Therefore cost was the real policy driver.[252]

Health of the Nation targets[251]

No.	Target	Target year	Movement towards target	Movement away from target
A1	Coronary heart disease < 65 years	2000	✓	
A2	Coronary heart disease 65–74 years	2000	✓	
A3	Stroke < 65 years	2000	✓	
A4	Stroke 65–74 years	2000	✓	
A5/B6	Cigarette smoking – male	2000	✓	
	– female	2000	✓	
A6	Blood pressure	2005	✓	
A7	Obese (%)	2005		✓
A8	Energy from saturated fat (%)	2005	✓	
A9	Energy from total fat (%)	2005	✓	
A10	Drinking – male	2005	No change	
	– female	2005	No change	
B1	Breast cancer 50–69 years	2000	✓	
B2	Incidence of cervical cancer	2000	No data	
B3	Incidence of skin cancer	2005	No data	
B4/5	Lung cancer	2010	✓	
B7	Giving up smoking in pregnancy	2000	✓	
B8	Cigarette consumption	2000	✓	
B9	Smoking 11–15 years	1994		✓
C2	Suicide all ages	2000	✓	
D1	Gonorrhoea – new cases	1995	✓	
D3	Conceptions under 16 years	2000	✓	
E1	Accidents under 15 years	2005	✓	
E3	Accidents ≥ 65 years	2005	✓	

Bovine spongiform encephalopathy (BSE) and Creutzfeldt–Jakob disease (CJD) had been a troublesome policy issue since the early 1990s. It was a matter for the wider department rather than the Executive, but it did eventually reach ministers, who made what were subsequently judged to be unwise public statements about the risks to public health. The medical division in particular was criticised in the subsequent inquiry.

In 1995 Calman (CMO for England) and Hine (CMO for Wales) launched their plan to improve cancer services.[205] It was about radically changing professional practice as well as building more capacity. Jobbing surgeons with a small volume of cancer cases had to go. It was not a question of the more a professional did the better he became, but rather that there was a minimum threshold below which competence could not be assured. Centres of excellence would be created for each of the major population centres, which would work closely with the cancer units based in the district general hospitals. There was much competition to become a designated cancer centre. This was the first time a major disease had been attacked from the centre, and it represented a major shift in focus for NHS management. They were now expected to deliver major change in how and by whom clinical services were provided.

Communications

Communication strategies featured quite strongly in Langlands' time. A communications team had been built up inside the Executive, in addition to the Department's press office in London. It tried to improve communications between the Executive and the NHS, and made some progress. This team started to protect the brand name 'NHS' and introduced the now familiar blue typeface, which was applied across the whole system. From 1992 the Executive published its own annual report, thus reinforcing its own identity at least within the NHS. A newsletter started to appear in staff-rooms and surgeries. However, by January 1996 the Executive was having an extended debate about reducing the volume of communication with the NHS.[375] Getting the balance right was a fine art.

NHS performance tables, which had been introduced in 1994, continued to roll off the production line, causing much comment in the process. Performance measures from the Patient's Charter had been increasingly tightened over time and were included in the tables. The waiting-times guarantee had changed from 2 years to 18 months. The Executive opened up the discussion with the BMA about the publication of clinical indicators and mortality tables.

Out in the wider world, the Executive's identity was inevitably swamped by that of Virginia Bottomley and her ministers. In the eyes of the public they ran the NHS, and the Major Government was in trouble. In April 1995, the *Health Service Journal* was forecasting that 'the end is nigh for Mrs Bottomley.' The picturesque image of her upholding her family traditions of marching towards gunfire in her determination to tackle the London problem would be a lasting one.[253]

In July 1995, Major reshuffled his cabinet and Bottomley moved across to the Heritage Department after six years at the Department of Health. Many who had worked with her wished her well. Her early-morning calls to officials might have been tiresome, but she clearly cared about the NHS. She more than anyone else had curbed (some would say smothered) the internal market and moved NHS management back to its public-sector roots. Her public image on leaving was poor: 'Mrs Bottomley is leaving the Department of Health not in triumph but as one of the most mocked and reviled figures in British politics. Whatever the eventual verdict of history, she stands in the opinion polls as an utter failure.'[254]

This was a harsh judgement. She was much better than that. She was good at projecting a caring image, which reflected her true feelings. She had taken the first decisive steps in sorting out the London problem, and even her opponents gave her credit for courage in tackling a problem that dozens of her predecessors had ducked. She promoted the wider public health agenda. She lost it in the detail she was so fond of quoting at every public appearance. She had to have every answer. If she had stood back a little and given the Executive the space she herself thought they needed, she might have achieved more and her image would have been better.

Stephen Dorrell takes over

Stephen Dorrell, Secretary of State, 1995–97

Stephen Dorrell was born in 1952, and was educated at Uppingham School and Brasenose College, Oxford.

He worked as a company director of his family industrial clothing company before becoming MP for Loughborough from 1979 to 1997 and for Charnwood from 1997. He was Parliamentary Private Secretary to Peter Walker, the Secretary of State for Energy from 1983 to 1987, Government Whip from 1987 to 1990, Parliamentary Under-Secretary of State for Health from 1990 to 1992, Financial Secretary to the Treasury from 1992 to 1994, Secretary of State for National Heritage from 1994 to 1995 and Secretary of State for Health from 1995 to 1997. He became Shadow Secretary of State for Education and Employment from 1997 to 1998, when he left the Shadow Cabinet and returned to the backbenches.

Stephen Dorrell returned to the Department of Health as Secretary of State in July 1995 with a reputation as a competent minister with a mind of his own and a belief in sound economics, including the PFI. The Labour Opposition judged him to be 'a very able guy, but he was sent in to play a dead bat.'[255] It was Alan Langlands who provided him with his written policy brief on taking up office.[256] Dorrell was a great believer in GP fundholding, which he regarded as 'the grit in the oyster' of the Conservative health reform.[257] As he took over, the Labour Party confirmed their intention, should they gain power, to abolish both the internal market and competition in the NHS. Dorrell was not by instinct a centraliser: 'No big business in the world, no other human activity, even including the military, any longer believes that the efficient way of delivering a defined objective is to concentrate all power at the centre.'[257]

The PFI process slowed down new capital investment as business cases had to be worked up with commercial partners. All NHS capital projects now had to have a PFI option. This was a costly and complicated process. Invariably the PFI plans had fewer beds than would have been provided under the old system. However, by 1995, when Dorrell took over, there were 20 major acute hospital developments under detailed negotiation.[256]

When the Labour Party was in opposition, Margaret Beckett as health spokesman was deeply opposed to the PFI.[259] This situation was to change as the election drew closer. As capital investment slowed, revenue became a problem again. From August 1996 revenue allocations were made directly by the Secretary of State. Deficits had begun to grow in many trusts, and GP fundholders started to overspend. Dorrell persuaded the Treasury to find another £25 million in December 1996 to soak up the financial consequences of winter pressures.

NHS Policy Board

NHS structure from April 1996[108]

Secretary of State
Accountable to Parliament for the NHS

NHS Executive and its eight regional offices
Co-ordinates local services within a single NHS

100 Health authorities (integrated DHAs/FHAs)
Cover both primary and secondary care
Primary expertise planning, administration and contracting for services
Accountable for the NHS within their districts
Responsible for the efficient use of resources
Challenge variations in treatment rates

The NHS Policy Board was re-jigged by Stephen Dorrell in November 1995 to accommodate the regional chairmen. Its terms of reference were by now explicitly focused on the management of the NHS. Its task was 'to provide a forum in which ministers and senior managers meet regional chairmen to consider current NHS management issues.'[220]

Its membership on inception was as follows:

NHS Policy Board, 1995[361]

Secretary of State for Health	Stephen Dorrell
Minister of State for Health	Gerald Malone
Parliamentary Secretary (Health)	Tom Sackville
Parliamentary Secretary (Community)	John Bowis
Parliamentary Secretary (Lords)	Julia Cumberlege
Permanent Secretary	Graham Hart
NHS Chief Executive	Alan Langlands
Chief Medical Officer	Kenneth Calman
Chief Nursing Officer	Yvonne Moores
Regional Chairmen:	
Trent	Keith Ackroyd
West Midlands	Bryan Baker
Anglia and Oxford	Stuart Burgess
South and West	Rennie Fritchie
Northern and Yorkshire	John Greetham
North Thames	William Staveley
South Thames	William Wells
North West	Don Wilson

A number of external members who had in one way or another played a significant role retired, including Professor Cyril Chantler, Sheila Masters, Peter Gummer and Kate Jenkins.

Dorrell's style was very different from that of Bottomley. He and Langlands met once a week (early on a Wednesday morning) on a one-to-one basis. They compared notes about the issues of the day, and Langlands got a lead when he needed it or when Dorrell wanted to give him one. They obviously met on other occasions at times of crisis, but this was the exception rather than the rule.

Langlands found Dorrell to be by far the easiest Secretary of State to work with. He describes him as 'a non-interventionist chairman, a big-picture chairman. He was interested in ideas and didn't get bogged down in detail.'[216] Nichol had also got on well with Dorrell when he was a junior minister. They had adjoining offices and 'often wandered into each other's offices late at night and chewed over the issues of the day and gossiped.'[257]

Dorrell quickly decided that there had been enough structural change and that it had not worked. 'If anything,' he concluded, 'the extent to which management change had actually changed the world as it was expressed in the surgery or the ward had been exaggerated.'[257] 'Management reform is yesterday's agenda,' he told party activists at a meeting in Cambridge. It was now time to start concentrating on improving services for patients. 'It was time,' he said, 'for managers to explain their decisions in language the public would understand.'[260]

This did not stop him demanding yet another cut in NHS management costs.[261] Overall the NHS had to find 5%,[262] including the trusts, who strongly resented what they regarded as an intrusion into their hard-won freedoms. They thought that it was for them to decide how much to invest in management. Their argument got them nowhere. Their 'M2' costs had to come down.

As a consequence, Dorrell had a hard time at the NAHAT Conference. Resignations were threatened, but most chief executives took the view that 'with a bit of luck there will be a change of government before they wake up to the fact that some of us are not implementing their cuts.'[262]

Langlands justified the management cost reduction on the grounds that the major reorganisation pressures were now over and some reduction was reasonable. This did not protect him and Dorrell from a furious onslaught from Karen Caines, the former civil servant who was now the Secretary of the Institute of Health Service Management (and, incidentally, married to Eric Caines, the former Director of Personnel in Nichol's team). Dorrell had, she said, 'derided the profession that had done much of the Government's dirty work.'[263] Dorrell backed off a centrally imposed target for the following year and tried to turn the cuts into good news: 'I am celebrating the success of management. Because it is more efficient, we have delivered that extra resource to patient care'. It was all a game of politics, with little rationale underpinning it except for the fact that the paper chase associated with the market was unnecessarily unwieldy. Langlands had to hand his own efficiency study, which suggested that a million pieces of paper could be eliminated, with a saving of £40 million.[264]

Labour managed to get in on the act by promising £100 million of savings in the bureaucracy without losing a single manager.[265] Tessa Jowell threatened that trusts which lost contracts with their local health authorities would close under a Labour government.[266]

In the middle of this the merger negotiations between NAHAT and the Trust Confederation developed into a messy public row, but eventually the NHS Confederation was created with Philip Hunt, a future Labour health minister, as its first director.

Computing problems again

The problems of introducing computing and information technology into the NHS continued to dog the Executive. All of the attempts to install major hospital systems had run into trouble and been delayed according to the National Audit Office. The Executive's own review had reported that even the most successful Hospital Information Support Systems (HISS) would cost an average of £2 million each over their ten-year lifespan.[269] In 1990 the Executive had become closely involved with Dr James Read, who was developing a coding and classification system for use in primary care. The Executive set up an NHS centre in Loughborough to develop the work, but left Dr Read owning the rights to distribute the codes once they had been developed. They paid Dr Read's company over £13 million. 'Put at its baldest,' said the *Health Services Journal*, 'it meant that an NHS official owned a company with an exclusive licence to sell crown copyright computer codes to the NHS.' 'It was,' said Rhodri Morgan MP, 'one of the most outrageous conflict-of-interest situations that I have ever come across.'[268] It was a mess that nearly cost the civil servant in charge of information management technology his job, particularly when it became known that the contract with Read had a non-disclosure clause.

When Langlands was challenged by the PAC in March 1998, he had to admit that it had all been a ghastly mistake by his predecessor 'at a time when the climate was very different.'[269]

Information technology was a problem principally because the speed with which it was developing was far too fast for the slow-moving NHS. The level of investment was preposterously small and the system was totally intolerant of mistakes. As Roy Lilley put it, rather unkindly, 'the NHS was a paper-driven slum when it should be an IT showcase.'[270]

However, Research and Development was significantly better targeted and managed by 1996, following the creation of a single national budget funded from a special levy on all health authorities.

A Service with Ambitions

In November 1996 Dorrell launched yet another NHS plan, this time called *The National Health Service: a service with ambitions*.[208] It had been crafted by a team from the Executive led by Alasdair Liddell, the Director of Planning, and it contained a well-argued case for a publicly funded NHS. It committed the Conservatives to an NHS available to everyone on the basis of need, regardless of the ability to pay: 'Hard choices would be required, but these were best made locally rather than nationally.' A primary care-led NHS was the way forward, supported by a well-informed citizen. It argued the case for a major investment in information technology, a more skilled workforce and knowledge-based decision making. The plan was full of good ideas, many of which were developed in the coming years as part of Labour's modernisation agenda. The other significant shift was away from a policy dominated by notions of equity towards one that took as an objective 'a high-quality, integrated health service which is organised and run around the health needs of individual patients, rather than the convenience of the system or institution.'[208]

Primary care reform

In December, Dorrell followed up with a White Paper on the reform of primary care, entitled *Primary Care: delivering the future*.[271] Health authorities were to be given the responsibility for raising standards and improving access to primary care. The salaried GP was to become a real option, and the GP's semi-detached relationship with the NHS was to end. The NHS pension scheme was to be opened up to practice staff for the first time, and nurse prescribing was to be extended. The manner in which primary care funds were allocated was to change to more closely match need, and a new suite of primary care performance measures was promised. The response from the profession was reasonably warm, although they were expecting a large pay award to accompany the changes. Mental health also got a Green Paper that proposed building new partnerships between health, local government and the independent sector.

However, it was all looking too late. As the election of 1997 approached it looked increasingly likely that Labour would win. Health authorities and trusts began to take a close interest in what the other parties had in mind for the NHS. To see how it looked in April 1997 see the table opposite.[272]

Although in their different ways all of the political parties promised to save the NHS, Langlands and his team had to face up to the prospect of a total reversal of much of what they had been pursuing. Everything slowed down. The NHS had become a political football.

By this stage the NHS was approaching another crisis. The workload was increasing and deficits were accumulating again. Elective surgery had doubled between 1981 and 1995 and was continuing to increase. Medical emergencies had risen by 13% in 1994–95 and no one was quite sure why. The winter of 1995–96 was to prove even worse, with an increase of 37%.[273] Length of patient stay in hospital had been falling for a generation or more,[208] and the hospital sector was beginning to struggle with the combined pressures to deal with waiting lists and cope with increased medical emergencies. Beds were at times in very short supply as the system soaked up surges of demand with only very limited recovery time. The slack had been largely squeezed out of the system. The NHS was hitting 2.25% on the Efficiency Index, compared with the long-running average of 1.5% per annum.[256] Langlands had admitted on the *Today* radio programme that he had never known the service to be under such pressure before. The story ran all day, much to the discomfort of Dorrell. A few days later Langlands showed Dorrell the letters that he had received thanking him for telling it as it was. 'When did you last get 200 letters after a radio interview?' Langlands asked him.[216]

The early months of 1997 saw the enforced departure of a number of chief executives as politicians talked toughly about performance. Chris Smith, the Labour spokesman, also made it plain that 'managers' jobs were on the line' if they did not deliver his party's performance targets.

Political party plans for the 1997 election

Labour	Conservative	Liberal Democrat
Funding		
Raise real-term spend every year	Raise real-term spend every year	Spend at least £540 million more on the NHS by increasing tax on cigarettes
Encourage PFI	Encourage PFI	
Internal market		
To be scrapped	Market to develop	Move to three-year contracts
3–5-year agreements to replace contracting		
Fundholding		
To be scrapped	To be developed with super-surgeries and enhanced Cottage Hospitals	GPs who wish to do so to be allowed to manage their own affairs
To be replaced by GP commissioning involving other disciplines		
Community care		
Royal Commission on long-term care	Stop closure of long-stay hospitals until adequate community alternatives are in place	Raise threshold at which older people contribute to long-term care
	Partnership scheme for funding long-term care	Halt bed closures for six months
Boards		
To be made more accountable	No change	Move to elected local bodies with half of the members coming from the local population
Managers to be held to account		
Pay and manpower		
National system with local flexibility	More doctors and specialist nurses	End local pay
		NHS pay review body
		More doctors and nurses
Public health		
Public health minister to be appointed	Keep *Health of the Nation*	Ban tobacco advertisements
		Free eye and dental checks to be reinstated
Quality		
New Patient's Charter	More league tables	Independent National Inspectorate
Waiting Lists		
Extra 100 000 patients to be treated	NHS already treating 1 million extra patients each year	Six months maximum wait within three years
No waiting for cancer surgery		

In May 1997, Ken Jarrold announced his decision to leave his national post, despite having two years to run on his contract, and to move back into the NHS as Chief Executive of County Durham District Health Authority. He had not enjoyed his time at the centre. There was much speculation about his reason for leaving, but the *Health Services Journal* captured the most common view – that the move back into the NHS represented a definite gain for NHS management.

The Civil Service meanwhile got down to its traditional job of preparing two very different briefs for a newly elected incoming government. One was about taking forward and developing existing policies, while the other was about demolishing the internal market that had been so painfully constructed over the previous eight years. This was a job for the professional civil servants. It required intellect without passion.

1997: Labour takes over

Frank Dobson, Secretary of State, 1997–99

Frank Dobson was born on 15 March 1940, and was educated at Archbishop Holgate Grammar School, York and the London School of Economics.

He worked in the Headquarters of the Central Electricity Generating Board from 1962 to 1970, for the Electricity Council from 1970 to 1975, and was Assistant Secretary, Office of Local Government Ombudsman for England from 1975 to 1979. He was a Camden Borough Councillor from 1971 to 1976 and Leader of the Council from 1973 to 1975.

He became Member of Parliament for Holborn and St Pancras in May 1979. Between 1982 and 1997 he held positions as opposition spokesman in the Departments of education, heath, energy, employment, transport and the environment. He was Shadow Leader of the House of Commons from 1987 to 1989. He was Secretary of State for Health from 1997 to 1999, when Alan Milburn took over. In 1999 he stood against Ken Livingston as Mayor of London and lost.

Labour won by a landslide. Langlands was at home in Yorkshire waiting for an announcement about the cabinet. Graham Hart, the Permanent Secretary, was in London waiting to induct the new Secretary of State into his office. It was to be Frank Dobson. He had been Shadow Health Secretary in the 1980s and had taken a close interest in the problems of the NHS in London. He was received by Graham Hart and presented with his brief: 'Two feet thick with a summary of what his party had promised to do.'[191] He was astonished. The truth, at least according to Alan Milburn, was that when they came into power Labour had no detailed plans about what to do about the NHS other than to reverse the Conservative reforms.[255]

Two days later the new ministerial team gathered in the Secretary of State's office in London. The arrangement of the chairs was different from that in Dorrell's time, which seemed symbolically to signal change. Everyone was euphoric. Langlands watched it all, wondering whether he would still have a job at the end of the day. At 10.00 a.m. they were summoned to Downing Street. The Prime Minister wanted to talk about health. Langlands joined the ministerial team. He had never met Tony Blair before. Blair looked Langlands straight in the eye and said 'What do you think about our policy on primary care? Should we be getting rid of fundholding?'[216] Langlands' response was the product of many appearances before the House of Commons committees: 'If it says so in the manifesto, yes you should.' Langlands was to see much of Blair in the coming months as the Labour Party tried to get to grips with the NHS. Blair had set the tone while in Opposition when he threatened to send hit squads into poorly performing parts of the NHS.[273]

Dobson was a challenging Secretary of State. He chose as his political adviser Simon Stephens, who had some experience as an NHS manager. Alan Milburn and Tessa Jowell became his Ministers of State, with Baroness Jay looking after Health in the Lords. An early concern of Dobson was to find out who was in charge:

> I had a very strong view that nobody was in charge and it needed to have people put in charge. . . .The theory of the establishment of the Executive might have been sound, the only thing was, it didn't really exist in practice, and all sorts of basic tasks were simply not being done. There were allegedly standards for breast cancer care and cervical screening with one trust monitoring 12 others. It was demonstrably not working.[191]

Langlands and his team soaked up the pressure and were constantly in London rather than at their headquarters in Leeds.

Dobson had little regard for the Executive Team, some of whom he described as 'essentially derivative, second-rate, basically incompetent.'[191] However, he did grow to respect Langlands, although he knew that he was asking him to demolish policies that he must have believed in when they were introduced. He thought that Langlands needed a deputy to 'ramrod' change from the centre.

Alan Milburn took a similar view: 'You had to inject some steel into the spine of the NHS. When we came in in 1997 there was no spine, it was crumbling, there was neglect and a huge problem of resources.'[255]

Dobson inherited an NHS that was still in a state of crisis. Cash remained short, and many health authorities were again accumulating large underlying deficits. Langlands did not disguise the scale of the problem. Another injection of cash was going to be essential to meet winter pressures. Waiting lists were soaring despite the fact that during the period from October to December 1997 the NHS had treated more patients than at any other time in its history. Dobson quickly redefined the waiting-list targets to be delivered within the life of the Parliament, but dismantling the whole of the internal market was more challenging. The plan for the new NHS when it emerged in December 1997 had something in it for everyone. It was full of exciting promises such as 'Everybody with suspected cancer will be able to see a specialist within 2 weeks.' Excellence was guaranteed for all patients, as was 'a new information superhighway' to give patients more choice about where to be treated. Its title, *The New NHS: modern, dependable*,[209] picked up the Blair theme of 'modernisation', which was softer than 'change' or 'reorganisation.' The new NHS would be 'based on partnership and driven by performance.' The split between purchasers and providers, a cornerstone of the

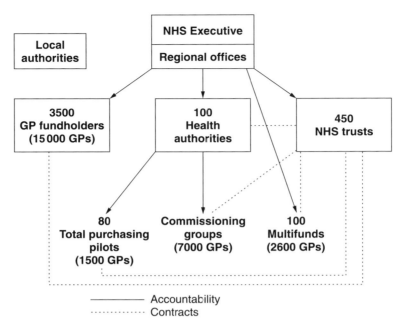

Figure 5.2 The old NHS: pre-1998.

Conservatives' internal market, would remain. Fundholding was changed into a network of primary care groups (PCGs), giving GPs control over the £35 billion health budget. This sustained primary care purchasing, but with larger groupings with a multi-disciplinary membership. It was a clever way out of fundholding. PCGs would have, for the first time, a unified budget for primary and secondary care and could swing investment across the old divide. Trusts remained *in situ*, but with instructions to collaborate rather than compete. Chief executives were to have a statutory responsibility for quality. A raft of new quality initiatives was launched, including the National Institute for Clinical Excellence (NICE) and the Commission for Health Improvement (CHI). Health action zones (HAZ) with dedicated funding were to be created to stimulate local partnerships to improve the health status of deprived communities. As *The Times* put it, the aim was 'to break down the Berlin Wall between health and social care.'[274]

It represented a ten-year plan to renew and improve the NHS through what was called evolutionary change rather than organisational upheaval. These were soothing words for hard-pressed managers, but they masked what was to become one of the most radical reorganisations of all, as primary care groups assumed their new roles and managers changed jobs once again. The contrast between the old and the new structure was portrayed rather simplistically (as shown in Figure 5.2) in the presentation packs that were distributed to all senior staff to help them to explain the changes to others.[209]

Langlands left the politicians to announce the new plan (which in any case Dobson judged to be his job),[275] and the NHS Executive deliberately kept quiet in the days after publication, 'to allow time for the message to sink in.'[276] Langlands was even inclined to wear a hair shirt with a comment to a manager's conference

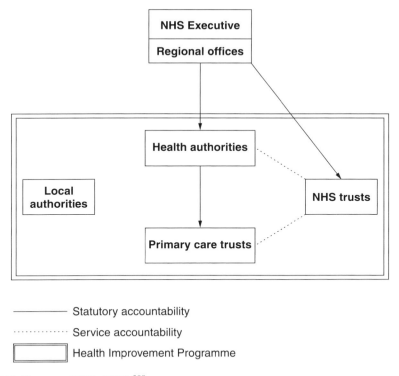

Figure 5.3 The new NHS: 1998.[209]

about the Conservative reform programmes: 'a small group of us, a couple of thousand people, took off and left everybody else in their wake.'[276]

The truth was that the politicians and their advisers had not only written the plan themselves, but they were also determined to have control over its implementation. They did not have sufficient confidence in the Executive to leave it to them.

They were also in power after a very long spell in opposition. Alan Milburn captures the mood of the time:

> There was a sense of expectation about us being able to put the NHS right. . . . when you come into Government having been out for so long you want to put it right, you want to get on with it, and get your hands dirty and get your sleeves rolled up and get on with the job.[255]

Talk about rationing was still a taboo subject but Dobson himself, who understood the need to prioritise services, intervened directly when Viagra came on the market. Although it is a drug for treating impotence, many worried that it would become a lifestyle drug and put an enormous strain on NHS drug budgets. Dobson insisted on limiting its availability. It was a classic piece of national rationing, and the NHS rather liked it. The Secretary of State could make all the tough decisions in future.

Labour and London

Like his immediate predecessor, Dobson found himself quickly embroiled in the plans to change the NHS in London, in which in any case he had taken a close personal interest while in opposition. The Bottomley decision to effectively close Bart's Hospital was still being resisted, and Dobson wanted a different solution.

Dobson was very clear why the process of change had been so difficult. It was, he claimed, 'a lunatic policy of closing beds and hospitals. As the beds went down the waiting lists and delays went up. If you are doing something which is as diametrically opposed to common sense, the odds are you will find it difficult to bring about change.'[191] He was also much exercised about the problems of recruiting and retaining staff in the capital.

Dobson asked two more leading doctors to review the plans for London. Sir Leslie Turnberg, a former president of the Royal College of Physicians and his panel thought that primary care in the capital was woeful, and were worried about keeping up the standard of specialist practice.[277] Sir Terence English, a former president of the Royal College of Surgeons, urged Dobson to proceed with some degree of specialty rationalisation and concentration. One of the principal political problems was the future of Harefield Hospital, which Magdi Jacoob had built into a cardiac centre with an international reputation. The plan proposed to close Harefield and move the cardiac unit to St Mary's. The last thing Dobson wanted was a public fight with one of London's heroes. He called Jacoob in to see him. Jacoob did not want to see Harefield close, but he saw the potential benefits to cardiac surgery if an expanded unit with new facilities, including state-of-the-art laboratories, was developed at St Mary's. He agreed to go along with the plan. For this Dobson considered him to be a saint.[191]

Dobson began the process of re-working the plan for London yet again, based on the advice that he had received from Turnberg and English. Bart's was eventually turned into a cardiac and cancer centre as part of the new, invigorated London Hospital Group. It was at this point that Dobson decided to opt finally for a single London Regional Office.[275]

Sir Christopher Kelly, Permanent Secretary, 1997–2000

Sir Christopher Kelly was born in 1946, and took an MA at Trinity College, Cambridge. His early Civil Service career was primarily in the Treasury. Later he was Director of Fiscal and Monetary Policy from 1994 to 1995, and Permanent Secretary at the Department of Health from 1997 to 2000. He has been Chairman of the National Society for the Prevention of Cruelty to Children since 2002.

In 1997, Graham Hart retired as Permanent Secretary. He and Langlands had worked well together, but politicians were already beginning to question the need for two posts. As Dorrell put it, 'Hart, Langlands and I got on perfectly well together. Pretty well any system can be made to work if people know what has to be made to work, and there was a willingness to try to do so. Was it a sensible way to run a whelk store? Probably not!'[257] Hart was replaced by Chris Kelly, who found himself with a job that was inevitably marginalised by the well-established Chief Executive, the CMO and the Secretary of State's political advisers. As Dobson put it, 'he did not have a real job to do.'[191]

The Hospital Beds Inquiry

Dobson's strong views about bed closures led him eventually to demand a national beds inquiry, which he announced to much applause at the Labour Party Conference in Blackpool in 1998.[213, 278] He had listened to the arguments about reduced length of stay, day surgery and modern primary care, but remained unconvinced. He read in his papers every day about bed shortages, medical emergencies waiting on trolleys and cold surgery being cancelled due to lack of beds. Inner London, which Dobson knew best, had lost over 1000 beds between 1991 and 1996. In July 1998 he used a statutory directive (for only the second time in the history of the NHS) to stop Salford and Trafford Health Authority proceeding with plans to rationalise paediatric services.[279] The Hospital Beds Inquiry was undertaken by Clive Smee, the senior health economist in the Department of Health.

It was a complex issue, but a slow decline in beds in the acute hospital sector had been deeply embedded in national policy for years. However, surges in medical emergencies had put the remaining capacity under serious strain. All over the country plans to rationalise services were put on hold.

When the Inquiry reported, in February 2000, it confirmed that the number of beds had declined from 480 000 when the NHS was first set up to 190 000 in 1998. However, this reduction was more than offset by a shift towards day-case treatment and shorter lengths of stay. Activity was continuing to rise sharply.

Hospital beds[280]

Year	Acute	Geriatric medicine	Maternity	Mental illness	Learning disability	Total
1970	162 000	57 000	22 000	123 000	59 000	423 000
1980	146 000	55 000	18 000	87 000	49 000	355 000
1990–91	117 000	46 000	14 000	55 000	23 000	255 000
1998–99	107 729	28 697	10 398	35 692	7491	190 006
1999–2000	167 218	27 862	10 203	34 173	6834	246 290
2000–01	107 956	27 838	9767	34 214	6316	186 091
2001–02	108 535	28 047	9812	32 783	5694	184 871

The Government decided that the long-term trend had to be arrested. The answer lay in the provision of more acute beds and in the development of new intermediate-care beds, which would allow the existing acute beds to be used for their intended purpose. A significant expansion in NHS beds was planned for the first time in decades. By 2001–02 the number of acute beds had risen by 1500 compared with 1999–2000.[280]

Private Finance Initiatives

The money to fuel a hospital building programme would have to come from public/private partnerships, to which the Labour Government was an enthusiastic convert. Margaret Beckett's trenchant rejection of this option while in opposition had been overwhelmed by economic reality.[259]

In February 1998 the Government announced 11 new PFI schemes with a total value of £750 million. Public-sector capital, at least for new schemes, melted away. Both Dobson and Milburn took a lot of flak from the trade unions. Eventually, around 18 months later, they reached an uneasy compromise which meant that NHS staff did not automatically transfer to private employers. This calmed things down, but the problem was to return time and time again. The unions were not persuaded that the PFI was right for the NHS, and they were supported in this view by others on the left of the political spectrum, including Will Hutton, who said as much in an NHS Fiftieth Anniversary lecture.[281] In another lecture in the same series Graham Hart, the former Permanent Secretary, argued about the application of the PFI policy to the health sector. At the end of 2000 Milburn was still stoutly defending the PFI policy at the Health Select Committee.[282] The issue would not go away.

Accountability and the Fallon Inquiry

In January 1999, Dobson was presented with the report of the Fallon Inquiry[210] which had been sitting, mainly in public, for the previous 18 months.

In September 1996, a patient in Ashworth High Security Hospital in Liverpool had escaped while on an escorted visit into town. Stephen Dagget had managed to get to France, but returned a few weeks later and presented those who interviewed him with a dossier about life at Ashworth. He alleged drug dealing, pornography, attempted murder, corruption, incompetence and, most worrying of all, stories about a young female visitor who had spent a great deal of unsupervised time with two patients with a background of violent paedophilia. Much of the story was old news but had been kept quiet by the authority. This was a particularly sensitive inquiry for the Department of Health, because the three high-secure special health authorities reported directly to them at the time when the alleged incidents took place.

Langlands had given evidence to the Inquiry in public on 1 December 1997. He was well briefed and represented by counsel. In his evidence he said that he was accountable for the NHS Executive but not for the NHS. Asked where he fitted in the accountability chain, he responded:

> I had no formal line management relationship. You were right in identifying me at the beginning of this discussion as the Chief Executive on the NHS Executive. That is not the same as being the Chief Executive of the NHS. The NHS is made up of a series of statutory authorities, essentially about 100 health authorities, some special health authorities like the SHSA, and about 420 trusts.[210]

'He was', he explained, 'the Secretary of State's principal policy adviser for the NHS and accounting officer for the NHS budget.' In this latter capacity he could remove the accounting officer status from a chief executive but could not sack him or her. He went on to say 'Neither I nor the regional director can hire and fire the chief executive of a health authority, a special health authority or an NHS trust. That is the job of the chairman, with the assistance of the other non-executive members of the Board.'[210] In practice, of course, one would almost certainly lead to the other. Langlands had a big stick behind his back, and most chief executives knew this.

Langlands saw no real problems in making this complex system work. If he saw things going wrong he could intervene on behalf of the Secretary of State, but to have a line relationship with 530 chief executives was, in his view, simply impracticable, even with eight regional directors.

This did not sit comfortably with the earlier Statement of Accountabilities, which said that he was in charge of the NHS. However, it did accurately reflect the true legal position. The Statement was another episode in the long-running charade surrounding the role of the Chief Executive.

The conclusions of the Fallon Inquiry were unusually robust on the question of accountability.

> Who, we asked ourselves, is accountable when a whole system is flawed and to whom? We searched for some principles that might assist us in judging fairly those individuals who were working within such a system. We did not find any. Instead we found confusion and ambiguity.

The ambiguity starts at the top. The NHS Executive led by Sir Alan Langlands is not in charge of the NHS in the accepted sense of that expression. The NHS Executive is part of the Department of Health. The Chief Executive and his staff are civil servants. They have no line of direct accountability for the actions and conduct of NHS field authorities.[210]

Frank Dobson promised a review of accountability, but if one was undertaken it never saw the light of day. The extraordinarily complex network of relationships, power and influence at the top of a very large public service was set to continue. Nobody had any real incentive to change matters. Chairmen liked the idea of being accountable to a minister, who in turn liked the ability to politically manage decision making in the NHS. The system also protected the Civil Service status of those on the Executive. They appeared nowhere in the chain of accountability. It was a non-issue except for those who wanted the NHS to have a real head office with the power and authority to get a grip on an increasingly complex and crisis-ridden organisation.

Appointing managers

Dobson did, however, want more of a hand in the appointment of chief executives in the NHS. He wanted the best managers in the toughest jobs, which meant some degree of national control over appointments. He favoured the French system of public administration, with its emphasis on national training and career development. He was scathing in his criticism of traditional methods of selection by individual authorities: 'You can get a person appointed to run a major trust on a sleepy afternoon who is a dumbo.'[191] The best managers could be used as firefighters to run failing or badly managed trusts.[283] His advice was later followed by Milburn with regard to the selection of chief executives for the strategic health authorities. The centralisation nut had been given another twist.

Community care

The problems surrounding community care in England had, as promised, been hived off by the Government to a Royal Commission that was given a year to report. By this stage the NHS had very little long-term care capacity of its own and was applying the eligibility criteria quite strictly. By this stage, too, ministers had given in to pressure for national criteria. Local authorities were struggling to fund the demands they faced for packages of care in both the residential sector and the home. Elderly patients began to block hospital beds as they waited for the community package to be assessed and funded. The Commission reported in March 1999[284] with a majority report. This report reflected the widespread concern about means testing for access to long-term care and the wide variations in standards in the residential and nursing-home sector. Some people, they said, faced impoverishment before they received any help.

The majority of the Commission wanted all care, including personal care such as washing and feeding, as well as nursing care, to be free. The minority argued that this would be too expensive and in any case would benefit mainly the better off.

The Government's answer was to make all nursing care free and to set up a National Care Standards Commission. These steps eased but did not solve the problem. When the new Commission did eventually set mandatory standards it was forced to change them to advice, in the face of a potential collapse of the nursing-home sector. NHS trusts were later required to assess patients' continued eligibility for NHS care prior to discharge from hospital.

Our Healthier Nation and our new NHS

In March 1998, the new Government and its first Minister for Public Health, Tessa Jowell, published its Green Paper on public health, *Our Healthier Nation*.[211,285] It was, as John Appleby put it, 'a politically modified version of *Health of the Nation*.'[286] The policy was essentially the same, but the words were different. Out went low incomes and in came poverty. The essential facts were as startling as ever to a first reader. The death rate of unskilled men from lung cancer was four times greater than that of the professional classes, and the unskilled had a life expectancy that was five years less. The plan opted to stick with health targets, like its predecessor, but one target in particular was to dominate much of the NHS agenda for the next five years. This concerned waiting times for non-emergency surgery. Langlands and his team were stuck with an election promise to cut both the numbers waiting and the time that patients waited. When Dobson arrived in office the lists were going the wrong way. As at December 1997 there were 1 262 000 people on the inpatient lists, a 14% increase on the previous year. Worse still, the numbers of patients at the end of the list had doubled to 46 000, and over 1000 patients, the majority of whom were in London, had broken through the Patient's Charter barrier. All of this was despite the fact that the NHS was busier than ever with a volumetric increase in the number of non-urgent operations performed and a continued increase in the number of emergency admissions.

Admission to hospital in England[280]

Year	Emergency (x 10³)	Growth (%)	Elective (x 10³)	Growth (%)	Day-case rate (%)	Total (x 10³)
1996–97	3621	–	4565	–	60	8186
1997–98	3753	3.7	4655	2.0	62	8408
1998–99	3873	3.2	5093	9.4	64	8965
1999–00	3911	1.0	5160	1.3	65	9071
2000–01	3967	1.4	5277	2.3	66	9244
2001–02	3986	0.5	5314	0.7	67	9299

Dobson knew how sensitive this issue was and demanded action. Everyone knew it was not the numbers on the list that mattered but the time people waited, but the press loved the absolute numbers, as did the Conservative opposition, which was slowly emerging from the election defeat under its new leader, William Hague.

Because focus groups and independent polls kept telling the Labour leadership that this was their prime measure of success or failure, waiting-list management and reduction were to dominate strategic thinking at the centre and the lives of NHS managers for years to come. Although many clinicians welcomed the extra cash that it brought both into their part of the service and into many surgeons' and anaesthetists' pockets, they continued to object to the principle of time, rather than clinical priority, being the key determinant of treatment. Some developed their own points systems for determining clinical priority.[287]

Labour and NHS investment

Tony Blair and Gordon Brown, the Chancellor of the Exchequer, had honoured their promise to inject new money into the NHS with a three-year settlement of £21 billion (£18 billion for England) in July 1997. The new investment was widely applauded, for as Rudolf Klein put it, it represented a generous birthday present.[288] It was an increase in real terms of 4.7%. The trouble was that it had done little to solve the underlying problems. It was rather like a summer shower in the desert. Dobson had argued hard for increased investment, but the key word in the early years of Gordon Brown's term as Chancellor of the Exchequer was prudence, particularly where public spending was concerned. There was nearly a breakthrough in the run-up to the first party conference after the election. Langlands recalls being with Tessa Jowell when Dobson walked in and told him to prepare himself for a meeting with the Chancellor. He was to go on his own without a minister. The following morning he walked round to the Treasury to meet Gordon Brown and Alistair Darling, the Financial Secretary to the

Treasury. It was a somewhat heated and confrontational meeting during which Langlands attempted to both explain the current position and argue for increased investment. They left him with nine questions to answer by the following day. It was all to be handled in the strictest of confidence. Langlands worked through the night with Peter Garland, an experienced civil servant who had become the Regional Director for the North and Yorkshire, until an answer was ready. When it arrived at the Treasury the official who read it was appalled. 'I cannot give this to the Chancellor,' he explained, 'it's too hard-hitting, it's too clear, it's too everything. You cannot talk to the Chancellor of the Exchequer like this.'[216]

This was a cold, hard presentation of the facts, not a piece of smooth, polished briefing of the kind expected of a Permanent Secretary.

There the matter lay, and Langlands awaited the Prime Minister's party conference speech with bated breath. He was having dinner with Duke Hussey, Chairman of the BBC, when he received a call from the conference. It was all off, he was told, and there would be no announcement about more cash for the NHS. The NHS struggled on, but the press were now on the rampage. Day after day stories began to appear about the Third World NHS with cancer success rates on a par with those in Estonia. A national investment of only 6% of GDP in the NHS was 'a very low figure for an advanced nation,' said *The Times*.[258] One pressure group alleged that patients were being starved to death. It was reported that a woman with throat cancer had had her operation cancelled four times and that as a result her tumour had become inoperable. Trolley waits in Accident and Emergency departments became commonplace.

The Chancellor found an additional £500 million in the March 1998 budget, but much of it was targeted at key political objectives, and waiting lists in particular. A further £20 million came from the Modernisation Fund in February 1999, and another £20 million in September 1999 for on-the-spot booking services. The NHS would struggle on with its underlying deficits and general cost pressures while at the same time launching high-profile national projects.

Some doubted whether the circle of NHS funding could ever be squared. In September 1999 a report by the Nuffield Trust and the Judge Institute of Management Studies at Cambridge told the Prime Minister that patient expectations would have to be managed and modernised.[289] Dobson did receive £250 million from the Treasury in November 1998 to deal with winter pressures, but it was only enough to patch over the underlying crisis.[217]

As Dobson left to fight the London mayoral election, he sent a handwritten note to Blair from his office in the Commons, warning him that the NHS needed at least an extra £2 billion in the following year if a serious crisis was to be averted.

Langlands and Dobson managed to build a working relationship, although Langlands had once had to show Dobson a draft of a formal permanent secretary's letter (the ultimate threat) to dissuade him from making a wholly inappropriate decision about the Blood Transfusion Service.

By this stage the Government was being regularly accused of spinning news about health. Every week it seemed that there was a new announcement about targeted allocations, some of which had already been announced in another form. Most crucially, the BMA claimed that the Government had exaggerated the 1997 investment of £21 billion by calculating it on a 1998–99 basis rather than the conventional year-on-year calculation, which would have produced a much lower headline figure of £8.6 billion. Cynicism and suspicion about the Government's honesty and intentions began to grow from this point onward.

Milburn takes over as Secretary of State

Alan Milburn, Secretary of State, 1999–2003

Alan Milburn was born in Birmingham in 1958, and was brought up in the mining village of Tow Law, County Durham. He was educated at Stokesley Comprehensive School and gained a BA in history at Lancaster University.

He was co-ordinator of the Trades Union Studies Information Unit in Newcastle, and was employed as Senior Business Development Officer in North Tyneside Council until his election to Parliament.

He was elected MP for Darlington in 1992 and quickly picked up a number of opposition front-bench briefs, including health and economic affairs. He was Minister of Health under Frank Dobson in 1998, and in the same year he became Chief Secretary to the Treasury. In 1999 he replaced Frank Dobson as Secretary of State for Health. He resigned from the Cabinet in 2003 to spend more time with his family. His partner is a practising psychiatrist.

Alan Milburn took over as Secretary of State in October 1999 to find an NHS still in crisis. On his second day in office he announced that he intended to proceed with radical reforms of the NHS and would take on any vested interests that tried to block modernisation.[290] He wanted to invest more, but he also wanted the NHS to change and become both more responsive to patients and more efficient. He was impatient with both the Department of Health and NHS management. He took the reins himself. During a visit to Farnborough Hospital in Bromley, he acknowledged that Dobson had done a brilliant job in laying the foundations of a modern NHS but, he said, 'Now is the time to build on these foundations by upping the pace of change. There will always be forces of conservatism who will resist change, but there is a modernising, radical agenda for the NHS that I am determined to pursue because the NHS cannot afford to stand still.'[291] He told the medical profession that they were in the last-chance saloon. If the NHS did not change, it would die. It was time, he said, for them to shape up and help him sort it out.[216] By the end of October he was speaking of the Government's determination to end the postcode lottery of care standards in social services, and proposing a sister organisation to NICE for social care. By November he was tackling the problem of poorly performing doctors. He had a very clear sense of what had to be done in order to modernise the NHS, and he knew at this stage that a major cash injection would be inevitable.[255]

He pulled together a Strategy Unit of outside experts to think about the future, led by Simon Stevens, his political adviser, and supported by a team of outsiders with Professor Chris Ham from the University of Birmingham as director. The Management Executive was not a body from which he expected to hear radical ideas. Despite this, Langlands himself had earned some personal respect from

Dobson, Milburn and Blair and had his contract renewed in the summer of 1999, with warm words from the Prime Minister. Although he got on reasonably well with the Labour politicians and Blair in particular, he was increasingly frustrated by Labour ministers' interventionist policies and their reliance on political and external advisers. The core policy work of the Department had been taken over by the political advisers and their outside experts. Langlands' Executive was being increasingly sidelined.

In September 1999, the NHS Executive had evolved to include a much stronger public health presence and a Director of Operations with a strong NHS operational background. It was still a large team of 17 people. Interestingly, the public presentation of the structure was at pains to point out that the CMO's accountability to the chief executive was only in respect of clinical governance, and had 'no bearing on his separate responsibilities as the Government's Chief Medical Officer.'

Meanwhile the NHS was exceptionally busy. Acute admissions had continued to increase, and pressure to reduce the waiting lists had pushed hospital-bed occupancy rates up to 85%.[280] For many hospitals, acute bed shortages became the norm and a state of crisis became routine.

The Government was not helped when one of its leading medical supporters, Lord Winston, the infertility specialist, gave an interview to the *New Statesman* in January 2000 following the treatment of his 87-year-old mother in the NHS.[293] After a long wait in casualty she had been admitted to a mixed-sex ward and was found lying on the floor shortly after admission. She caught an infection and had a leg ulcer. 'The Government had,' he said, 'been deceitful in its promise to abolish the internal market. It was no good,' he said, 'blaming everything on the Conservatives. Labour itself had not done enough.' This was a deeply embarrassing intervention from a Labour peer, and once again it forced open the bigger question of a step change in NHS funding.

The Royal Colleges and the Conservatives waded in behind Winston.

As the Millennium approached, the NHS along with other organisations prepared for the worst should its computers and embedded microchips refuse to perform. A special team at the Department of Health laboured for a year, ensuring that all of the necessary checks were made. The Millennium passed quietly enough, but the NHS was having a bad winter and January 2000 saw an unprecedented increase in the pressure on beds, and intensive-care beds in particular. There was not an empty intensive-care bed in the country, despite the fact that the Government had promised some months before to fund an extra 100 such beds. Langlands was at home in Yorkshire with three phones ringing. The first, his mobile, had the Number 10 Press Office wanting to know what was going on. The second was Alan Milburn demanding to know where the extra beds were, and the third was his office trying to warn him about the other two calls. To make matters worse, members of the press were camped outside his house demanding interviews. Was it true, they asked, that he was rather more in tune with Lord Winston than he was with Alan Milburn?[216]

Handling the intensive-care issue was more difficult. The Department did not know where the extra ITU beds were. As Langlands tried to explain to Milburn, 'because of shifts and staffing levels the designation of intensive-care and high-dependency beds was fluid.' 'That is completely unacceptable,' said Milburn. 'It may be,' replied Langlands, 'but it is the reality.'

NHS Executive, September 1999[292]

Alan Langlands
Chief Executive

	Liam Donaldson	Hugh Taylor	Yvonne Moores	Sheila Adam	Sir John Pattison	Alasdair Liddle	Colin Reeves	Ron Kerr	Regional Directors	
Post	Chief Medical Officer	Human Resources	Chief Nursing Officer	Health Services Director	R & D	Planning	Finance and performance	Operations	Eastern	Peter Houghton
Function	Clinical governance	Pay and employment Corporate affairs	Nursing quality Patient issues	Health services, including emergency care Ambulances Children Mental health Public health		Strategy and business planning Analytical services Information management and technology Communications Primary care		High secure psychiatric hospitals Procurement General management issues	London	Nigel Crisp
									North West	Robert Tinston
									North and Yorkshire	Peter Garland
									South East	Barbara Stocking
									South and West	Tony Laurance
									Trent	Neil McKay
									West Midlands	Stephen Day

Langlands had no choice but to pull together a team that started to ring around the country taking a count of ITU beds. The press kept up the pressure with the active support of the ITU specialists. On Saturday 15 January 2001, Langlands was told that he had to handle the matter, rather than ministers. Langlands suspects that the ministers knew what was going to be announced the following day. So he appeared at the television studios in Leeds amid the football and other sports results.

The next day, on the morning of Sunday 16 January, Blair appeared on the television programme *Breakfast with Frost*. Both he and the Chancellor had been promising more cash for the NHS in the second comprehensive spending review, but Blair went much further. He admitted that spending on the NHS 'was too low at the moment.' He pledged that if the economy performed as planned, within five years the NHS would be funded at the European average as measured by its share of GDP. This implied a huge increase of perhaps 25%, or £9 billion. The announcement was greeted with a mixture of applause, amazement and scepticism. The BMA described one of the most important announcements in the history of the NHS as yet another political ploy. John Appleby, at the King's Fund, said that the pledge was based on out-of-date statistics from the OECD.[294] The Treasury, which had clearly been bounced by Number 10, wriggled, arguing that the average itself would move during this period. They supported the increase but did not want to be committed in advance to huge uncapped investment. It was, they explained, a legitimate aspiration. But it was too late – the promise had been made.

Langlands resigns

Langlands and his team were not finding Milburn easy to work for. They had no doubts about his intelligence or his commitment to change, but he distrusted the Civil Service system and relied heavily on external advisers and his own instincts. He was very impatient with what he perceived to be a lack of progress in reforming the NHS. Public presentation became paramount as initiative after initiative was announced, usually with nationally targeted funding.

Langlands began to doubt whether he could ever build a relationship that would work. He started to think seriously about moving on after what had by then become a regular meeting between the Department and the ten leading doctors (presidents of the Royal Colleges and others). Milburn had sounded off about this being the last chance for the NHS. He told them that it was time they shaped up and helped him to sort out the mess. The doctors did not take this well. After the meeting, Professor Naran Patel, the President of the Royal College of Obstetricians and Gynaecologists, came up to Langlands and said, 'I doubt you will be able to work with him. Have you considered coming to Dundee as Principal of the University?'[216]

He hadn't, but he did, and that is what eventually happened. In February 2000 he announced his resignation, despite having almost four years of his contract left to run. He left on 14 February 2000, at the age of 47 years.

Langlands' resignation came as a surprise to many, including Milburn,[255] who was warm in his thanks and praise, saying that he had made a major personal and professional contribution to the modernisation of the NHS.[295] However, within 24 hours of the resignation stories began to circulate that Milburn was planning to call in nurses and hospital chiefs to run the NHS in an attempt to sideline Whitehall bureaucrats and speed up improvements.[296] Regional directors and many of their headquarters colleagues would no longer serve on the top board, as 'most of them had not been at the frontline of the NHS for at least 20 years, if at all, and had no experience of current practices.'[297] The idea of an NHS Modernisation Board with 15 hand-picked top professionals had its first outing,[296] but in such detail that it was obvious it had been in gestation for some time. Milburn, it was clear, was determined to personally oversee the next round of changes to the NHS.

For the complex chemistry at the top of the Department of Health to work, the Chief Executive and the Secretary of State have to be able to work together. It is little different from the need for the chairman of a company or public board to work together with the chief executive. When it does not happen, something has to give. Most Secretaries of State saw themselves as executive chairmen. This was a role they had positively blocked in the NHS itself, on the grounds that a balance of power between chairman and executive produced a healthier organisation than those in which the power was concentrated in the hands of a single person. Secretaries of State who stood back from the day-to-day business of the NHS were rare, Stephen Dorrell being perhaps the only recent example.

Although Alan Langlands had kept a low public profile, he was liked and respected by those with whom he worked closely. His leadership style was quiet, intelligent and considered. He was naturally close to the mandarins, from whom he received much respect. Solid, intelligent and dependable are words often used to describe him, rather than inspirational. Two anonymous managers, who perceived him differently, expressed it thus:

> I like Alan, but he does not inspire except on a one-to-one personal basis. He could improve his presentation, he could tell people what he is doing and where he thinks the NHS is going, and he could give clearer messages. Alan's leadership is not exciting – it is too low key and not positive enough.[298]

> Alan is almost a meta-leader. He is creating space for leaders in the NHS to work in. If people think what he has to do is ride up on a white charger, they are wrong. That is old NHS-think. Those who want him to be a leader in the old-style quasi-military fashion are not thinking in the new way. His job is creating space for leaders to lead. If it were not for him there would be much less space to lead in.[298]

The latter view fits more closely with Langlands' own perspective about leadership, which he had spelt out so clearly to the NAHAT conference just after his appointment had been announced:

> My emphasis is on leading change rather than leadership, and underlines the collective, complementary and multifaceted aspects of change. I want to play down leadership with its connotations of individualism and often one-dimensional heroism, and think more broadly.[202]

Milburn took his time deciding what to do next. In the interregnum Neil McKay, who had been appointed as Langlands' deputy in December 1999, acted up into the chief executive role. He was an experienced NHS manager and was widely respected in the north of England, where he had made his reputation as a cool but tough manager. For some time the politicians had thought that there was insufficient space for both a chief executive and a permanent secretary. Chris Kelly in his much-diminished role had never managed to secure the total confidence of ministers. At one point Milburn had sounded out Langlands about taking on the combined role. There must have been deep concern at such a prospect within the senior Civil Service. A decision was put on hold while the NHS Plan was finalised.

The NHS Plan: 2000

Despite any misgiving he might have had, Gordon Brown delivered in his March 2000 budget, ahead of his own spending review, a massive 7.4% increase in the following year and 5.6% in each of the following three years. At the end of this four-year period, expenditure on the NHS would have risen by 50% and be equivalent to 7.6% of GDP. By 2003–04 the NHS would be spending £63.5 billion, and this represented £2800 a year per household in the UK. Even the BMA found it difficult to argue when, together with the leaders of the health professions and the NHS, they were summoned to Downing Street shortly after the budget announcements. They were to hear that a new NHS plan was to be prepared, with their help, so that the new investment could be spent wisely. They had three months to prepare a plan.[299] Six working groups were formed, incorporating many of the leading players in the NHS and the health professions. The group also included Nick Ross the television presenter, Don Berwick, a leading American guru, and Bob Abberley, from UNISON. It was a clever and somewhat dramatic attempt to draw the NHS into preparing plans for its own future. Excitement levels were high as the work proceeded. The Government had regained the ground that it had lost with the health professions. A low-key announcement from the Treasury that Derek Wanless, the former NatWest Chief Executive, was to take a longer-term look at NHS funding was interpreted as another positive step. Gordon Brown was by now taking a close interest in the affairs of the NHS.

The Prime Minister was very closely involved, and chipped in with his own views as the discussion continued. He encouraged working with the private sector, but understood that boosting capacity in the private sector would accentuate problems for the NHS. He wanted to see the NHS working closely with Boots the Chemist, Specsavers and other private providers. He pressed for more progress on sorting out clinical support services, and was very enthusiastic about Patient Line TV, provided that it could be funded by the private sector.

The NHS Plan emerged in July 2000 and was trumpeted as representing the most far-reaching changes to the NHS since 1948. It heralded a ten-year programme of rebuilding and renewing the NHS. The NHS was to remain publicly funded and free at the point of need, but it was to be radically modernised. The plan was extensively leaked in advance of publication. It had been written by Milburn himself (literally, on his office computer)[255] together with a small group of political advisers and civil servants. Tony Blair and Gordon Brown had taken a close interest in the drafting of the plan. The NHS Executive was hardly involved at all, but all of the professions that had been represented in the working groups were required to sign up prior to publication, and they all did so.

The NHS Plan came with cash, with an immediate allocation of £600 million for the NHS in England, announced in the March budget, to be used for local hospital and GP funding, the new intermediate-care service and to remove the existing postcode lottery of care.[300]

The NHS Plan, 2000[378]

- Faster access for patients. Maximum 48-hour wait to see a general practitioner; maximum 3-month wait for an outpatient appointment and maximum 6-month wait for surgery by 2005.
- By 2005, every patient would be able to book hospital appointments and elective admissions.
- Patients whose operations had been cancelled on the day of surgery for non-clinical reasons were to be given another date within a month, or cash for private treatment.
- 100 new hospitals and 7000 extra beds by 2004.
- 7500 more consultants, 2000 more GPs, 20 000 extra nurses and 6550 extra therapists. There was to be a massive expansion in training places, including a further 1000 new medical school places and 1000 new specialist registrars. International recruitment was to be stimulated.
- A new consultant contract to be negotiated.
- PCTs were to be given an option to commission health and social care as a total package. Care trusts made possible if there was joint local agreement to do so.
- A National Performance Fund worth £500 million.
- An extra £9000 million investment in intermediate care.
- 20 diagnostic and treatment centres by 2004.
- Community Health Councils to be replaced by patient advocacy liaison services (PALS).
- A new national framework for co-operation between the private sector and the NHS.
- £300 million for new equipment, including 200 new CT scanners.
- £30 million for an NHS clean-up campaign.
- Private Finance Initiative to be expanded into primary care (LIFT programme).
- 500 one-stop primary care centres.
- UK Council of Health Regulators to oversee professional regulation.
- Modern IT systems in every GP surgery and hospital.
- The working lives and pay of NHS staff to be improved.
- Local government to scrutinise the NHS locally and have powers to refer contested service reconfigurations to an independent panel.

The summary above shows the major components of the plan, but there were many others – for example, the extension of the expert patient panel and a requirement that letters between clinicians about a patient's care should be copied to the patient as of right. The power to suspend or remove GPs from a primary care list was to be devolved to primary care trusts, and the right of consultants to appeal to the Secretary of State against dismissal was to be removed. It was full of tantalising detail.

With the plan came a new bureaucracy, including a Modernisation Agency charged with rolling out the plan. It would report to a Modernisation Board chaired by the Secretary of State. (In practice, the day-to-day accountability was to the Chief Executive.) The Department of Health would, it claimed, limit itself to performance monitoring and defending the interests of patients. It would start steering rather than rowing. This was a move designed to 'overturn traditional Whitehall bureaucracy and hierarchy, and the Modernisation Board would include the best modernisers in the NHS.'[296] A National Leadership Centre would be created within the Modernisation Agency. A National Clinical Assessment Authority to assess a doctor's performance after a complaint was to be set up. Non-Executive Board appointments would be made in future by a new Independent Commission, with regional commissioners who would subsume the residual role of regional chairmen, who would finally disappear. New performance systems were promised, with red, yellow and green categories, which became the prototype stars system, that promised good performers extra cash and more autonomy. Organisations that were judged to be failing would be offered advice, and if that did not work, the centre would intervene.

The initial reaction within the NHS was reasonably positive, as was most of the press comment. The BMA was more cautious and was expecting a major battle ahead about the new consultant's contract. Community Health Councils were shocked at their demise.

Performance management overload

The raft of targets in the plan was meat and drink to the new breed of performance managers who wanted to count everything and feed both the central bureaucracy and the star-rating systems. The worst thing that could happen to a performance manager was to be caught by surprise, particularly if the press got involved. They had to know everything just in case they received a call from the centre.

It is difficult to overstate how oppressive and demanding these targets became. They dominated local planning and resource allocation and squeezed the life out of local innovation. The National Service Frameworks (NSFs) for cancer, mental health, etc. had pretty much the same effect. A few targets would have been very powerful, whereas hundreds became destructive and lost most of their impact. Not filling in the paperwork properly became sufficient grounds for an organisation to lose a star grading, no matter how good services were on the ground. The power of the targets and the consequences of a failure added to the temptation either to massage the numbers or to interpret them in the most optimistic manner possible. The financial health of many trusts was disguised by, among other things, over-optimistic cost improvement programmes that everyone, including those at the centre, knew to be a fiction. The Audit Commission noted that waiting-list figures were being distorted by a number of trusts.[301] The information corruption in the NHS had become serious. The targets became the enemy rather than the goal. Spin was now working in reverse. If ministers demanded good news, they would have it.

Chapter 6

Nigel Crisp, 2000–

By now Alan Milburn had concluded that 'the Executive was nonsense. It was fiction.'[255] The decision to combine the posts of chief executive and permanent secretary was finally made in June 2000. The job was put out to open public competition. The new post was to carry responsibility for the whole Department's business covering public health, social care and the NHS, to reflect the increasingly close connection between policy development and implementation across the services. Milburn described the post as being 'at the cutting edge of health and social care reform.'[302] The Conservatives condemned the decision, which they said they would reverse when they came back into power. There was much speculation about potential candidates, and a number of Whitehall high-flyers were expected to apply. As in Mrs Thatcher's day, Downing Street had its own views about the qualities needed. According to *The Times*, Blair wanted a breath of fresh air by introducing an outsider, possibly from industry.[303] Among the leading NHS candidates were Neil McKay and Barbara Stocking (who went on to become the Director of Oxfam). The Civil Service selection panel, which included George Alberti, the President of the Royal College of Physicians, duly interviewed the candidates in October 2000, and the name of Nigel Crisp, the Regional Director of the NHS in London, was put to ministers and Downing Street for approval. He was a relatively unknown NHS manager with almost no public or professional profile outside London and Oxford. His style was described by those who knew him as quiet and unassuming, with a good mind for strategic thinking. One observer told the *Health Services Journal*, rather unkindly, that he was 'the John Major of the NHS. He is nice and harmless, but does not have a lot of spark or drive.'[304] 'Nigel who?' asked *The Daily Telegraph*. 'Funny you should ask. He is the new Chief Executive of the NHS.' John Cooper, a leading London manager, was judged by many to have got uncomfortably close to the truth when he said that 'charisma belongs to ministers and they don't normally want somebody to compete with them for the limelight.'[304]

However, Crisp had obviously done well in London, and his appointment was stoutly defended by Alberti. 'Crisp was,' he said, 'the best of a range of candidates both external and internal. I think people are underestimating Nigel. He's not just a safe pair of hands. He is a superb strategic thinker and that has come through already in London.'[304]

Sir Nigel Crisp, Chief Executive and Permanent Secretary, 2000–

Nigel Crisp was born in January 1952 and was educated at Uppingham and at Cambridge University. He spent five years working for the Halewood Community Council in Liverpool before joining Trebor, the sweet manufacturers, as production manager. In 1978 he became the manager of

---

Cambridgeshire Community Council, and in 1981 he joined the NHS as a Unit General Manager for learning disability services in East Berkshire. In 1986 he became Chief Executive of Heatherwood and Wrexham Hospitals and in 1988 he became Chief Executive of the Oxford Radcliffe NHS Trust. In 1997 he became the Regional Director in South Thames and later for the combined London offices. He became Chief Executive of the NHS in England and Permanent Secretary of the Department of Health in 2000.

Neil McKay stayed on for a while as Director of Operations, but eventually moved back into the NHS as Chief Executive of the large acute trust in Leeds.

The end of the Executive

In April 2001, Alan Milburn announced his intention to wind up the NHS Executive and its regional offices altogether. It was still the Secretary of State who made organisational decisions of this kind, although no doubt Nigel Crisp had been consulted. Milburn, who had previously been regarded as an arch centraliser, had decided to shift the balance of power in the NHS towards local communities and frontline staff. 'Milburn hands power to the frontline staff,' said the Department of Health press release.[305] Another major upheaval was under way. The organisation was about to be turned on its head. Health authorities and regional offices were to be swept away and the funding reinvested in frontline services. At least one estimate put the savings as high as £100 million a year. The announcement came on the day that the new Modernisation Agency was being launched at the Queen Elizabeth Conference Centre in London. Primary care trusts were to become the lead organisations for assessing need, planning and securing services for their local communities and improving their health. NHS trusts were to continue, and those that performed best would be rewarded with greater autonomy and freedom, an idea that was eventually shaped into Foundation status. On 1 April 2002, 95 health authorities were to be replaced by 28 strategic health authorities and they would be charged with strategic development and the performance management of both PCTs and trusts. However, they were left out of the revenue allocation loop which, they were later to argue, left them with little real power to shape events. In April 2003 the eight regional offices were to be replaced by four directors of health and social care. All headquarters posts would be based in Leeds or London. Crisp told his staff at the Department that 'we must take on those tasks which only we can do, and where we add value.'[306] The response from the NHS was mixed. Those in primary care[374] were excited at the prospect of extended powers, but as Mark Gould reported in the *Health Services Journal*, another view was that '1000 staff were to be sacrificed on the altar of change.'[307] Milburn came in for particular criticism about the fact that many staff who would be affected heard the news for the first time on the radio or read it in their morning newspapers. It did not sit well with the Government's promise to be a good employer. The decision had been leaked in advance. Cutting the bureaucrats made good headlines.[308]

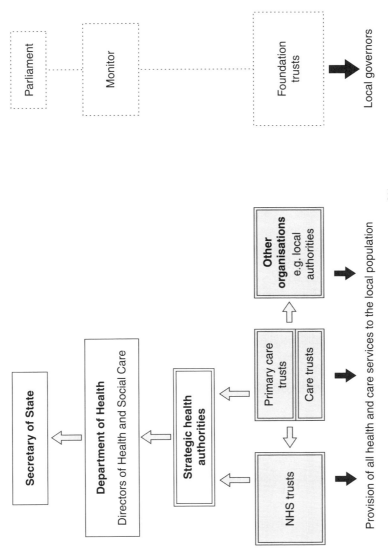

Figure 6.1 Organisation of the NHS in England as at 1 April 2002.[344]

Cynicism and spin

Public comment about the end of the Executive was muted, but the Government was facing a growing wave of cynicism about the public presentation of its policies and spin. Nicholas Timmins caught the prevailing mood in a piece in *The Financial Times* under the headline 'Spin doctors are killing the NHS', when he commented that 'historians may record that it was those who professed to love the NHS that killed it.'[309]

The new money was by now in place as promised, but the first tranche had been swallowed up by existing deficits and Government targets. The size of the underlying debt problem was substantial and was particularly focused in areas such as Bristol, Hertfordshire, Leeds and London, where difficult rationalisation decisions had been put off for years.

Timmins claimed that the conclusion that a model with much to commend it (i.e. a tax-funded service largely free at the point of need) was fatally flawed was wrong. It was the management of the project that had failed. 'The NHS might be destroyed by the Government's own hyping of expectations and excessive concentration upon structural rather than operational change.'[304]

'The danger was,' said Nigel Edwards, who at the time was acting as Director of the NHS Confederation, 'that politicians continue to promise in advance of the system's ability to deliver.'[319]

The Tories, while promising to match the Government's plan for spending on the NHS, also promised 'to take politicians out of the day-to-day management of the NHS' altogether.[311] The Liberal Democrats announced that they wanted to explore a Health Tax.[312]

By December 2001, Blair appeared to be backtracking on his promise to match European average spends on health except 'in the broadest of terms.'[313,319] Within only a matter of months, Milburn had decided that the four directors of health and social care were no longer needed. The strategic health authorities could stand perfectly well on their own and play their role at the local headquarters of the NHS.[315] Four of Crisp's most senior lieutenants who had successfully competed for these jobs against their colleagues were suddenly out of a job with little or no notice. They were privately furious, but nothing was said in public, for they were after all by this stage senior civil servants. No one dared to raise the issue of whether the Department in its new role had too many ministers.

Doctors and Labour

The medical and nursing professions had been relatively quiet during the early years of the Labour Government. Langlands and his team had done their best to keep them on side. The national clinical directors or 'medical Czars' as they were known had, it was thought, increased medical influence in the Department of Health, and extra money had been forthcoming. Milburn had attracted some criticism for his attack on the merit award system,[316] but other ministers and in particular Lord Hunt, the former Chief Executive of the NHS Confederation, had been warmer and more sympathetic. Lord Winston's outburst in January 2000 brought the professions' growing unease about the funding of the NHS and their own professional status closer to the surface. A series of independent reports had

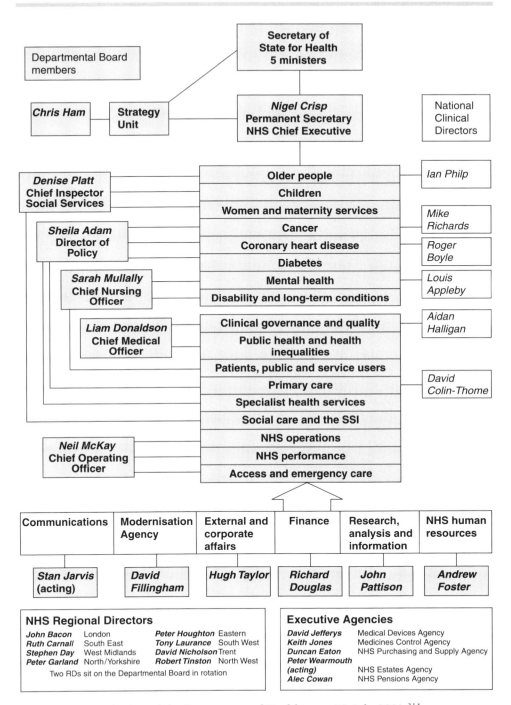

Figure 6.2 Organisation of the Department of Health as at 12 July 2001.[314]

criticised poor clinical performance by doctors. The General Medical Council seemed to be in the headlines every week as it dealt with those who had erred. Rodney Ledwood, 'the fastest gynaecologist in the south-east', was struck off in a storm of publicity for maiming many of his patients. Problems with the paediatric cardiac services in Bristol were causing a lot of public concern that led to an extended public inquiry chaired by Ian Kennedy. Health screening errors were being exposed more often, and were widely reported on each occasion. The error recall letter was built into routine practice. Problems with the national cervical cancer screening programme had been aired in 1998, when Alan Langlands had appeared before a PAC committee to respond to a particularly challenging National Audit Office report on the subject. Langlands had to admit his discomfort that national data were not available. The constant inability of the Chief Executive and ministers to provide Parliament with national data from a devolved NHS was a source of regular tension.

In January 2000, Harold Shipman, a general practitioner from Tameside in Greater Manchester, was convicted of murdering 15 of his patients, and another prolonged public inquiry was launched, chaired by Dame Janet Smith. In 1999 the scandal of retained organs after post mortem first hit the headlines. In the case of Alder Hey Hospital in Liverpool it became clear that organ harvesting went back decades, and that this was routine practice about which patients' relatives were rarely consulted. At around the same time the NHS fraudbuster was pursuing hundreds of doctors, pharmacists and opticians for the return of up to £36 million that had been allegedly defrauded from the NHS.[317] The medical profession was being hit from all sides and morale was low. In April 2001 the Government moved to prevent what *The Times* called the meltdown in the relationship between the Government and the professions. The mood of British doctors had, they claimed, reached boiling point.[303] The number of consultant vacancies was rising at the same time as workload was growing. Family doctors were threatening a one-day unofficial strike, and the BMA agreed to ballot its members about a mass resignation from the NHS. Peter Hawker, the Chairman of the BMA Consultants Committee, claimed that the NHS would collapse unless the next government stopped pushing up patient expectations.[318] To some extent the noise represented pre-election frenzy, but there was some substance to the BMA concerns. Morale among doctors was beginning to drop sharply as workloads increased inexorably and patients became more demanding. The doctors claimed that the public was also becoming disenchanted with the NHS, and MORI polls in December 2000 seemed to support this view. The number of people who were satisfied with the NHS had dropped from 72% in 1998 to 58% in 2000.[368]

Immediately after the election in June 2001, the BMA returned to the attack. In his opening address to the July BMA Conference, Dr Ian Bogle, a GP from Merseyside and leader of the BMA negotiating team, warned ministers that time was running out for the NHS.[320] 'Four years ago,' he said, 'the health professions had been enthused with optimism by Labour promises of regeneration. Four years on things could not get much worse.'[320] The fight about the new consultants contract rumbled on into the autumn of 2003, with regular threats of mass resignations.[321] Not for the first time, a government found itself embattled with the doctors whom it was relying on to lead a reformed NHS.

Redefining the NHS

In the period immediately after the 2001 election, the Labour Government spent a lot of time thinking about the reform of public services, which they had themselves put at the top of their manifesto agenda. Milburn and Blair started to talk about the importance of the public-sector ethos: 'Ask a teacher, a doctor, a nurse or a policeman why did they do their job and almost always it's about giving to others, not taking for themselves.'[310, 322] In a speech at the Royal Free Hospital, London, Blair promised continued investment (at least an average of 6.3% in each of the next three years), but only if it was accompanied by reform, and this included a new partnership with the private sector.[310] With this commitment came a warning that he 'would not flinch from the decisions and changes to deliver better public services, no matter how much opposition. If the changes are right, they will be done.'[310] 'We need every bit of help we can get,' said Milburn, 'to renew the NHS. The private sector could perform operations on NHS patients, run new stand-alone surgical units, extend PFI into primary care and manage the introduction of IT systems into the NHS.'[323] He followed this up in October by explaining that the central goal was 'making the public services user led, not producer or bureaucracy led.'[324] 'Public servants were,' he said, 'working flat out, but in a system that shrieks out for fundamental change.'[324] In November, Brown published the interim Wanless Report on long-term health funding.[325] This time Nigel Crisp and some of his colleagues had been directly involved in supporting an external expert, and one can detect their contribution in the detail contained in the report. Wanless had concluded that 'there was no evidence that any alternative financing method to the UK's would deliver a given quality of healthcare at a lower cost to the economy. Indeed other systems seem likely to be more costly.'[325] Despite this, it was clear that the NHS needed a much higher level of overall investment. As one Treasury official was reported to comment, 'We knew things were bad, but we did not know they were this bad.'[326] *The Sunday Times* waded into the argument with an 'Obituary to the NHS' which, it claimed, 'had long since ceased to be a revered icon.'[327] For the first time in public, at least, the Chancellor acknowledged that tax rises might be required to give Britain a world-class health service.[328]

During December, Blair, Brown and Milburn thrashed out a way forward. The shift away from Whitehall was to be accelerated. The NHS could no longer be run from Whitehall. 'We can't run the NHS from the centre any more. The command and control NHS no longer works,' explained a Treasury spokesman.[329] Downing Street brought in yet another external adviser, Adair Turner, the former CBI Director General, to review NHS management.[329] Gordon Brown, who had commissioned his own research into cost and quality variations within the NHS, was as appalled at the range as Mrs Thatcher had been in her day. Much of the variation, he believed, was down to poor management, which would have to be rooted out. In another move to put pressure on the system, Milburn announced in November that patients would in future be able to choose their hospitals, and that patients who had to wait more than six months in London could be treated in the private sector in the UK or elsewhere in Europe. Ministers signed an agreement that would take 1000 patients a year to Belgium for treatment.[330] In January 2002, in a speech to the New Health

Network,[331] Milburn announced that successful hospitals would be liberated from Whitehall by becoming foundation hospitals. 'The last great nationalised industry,' as Milburn described the NHS, 'was an untenable model for the twenty-first century. We must redefine the NHS from a centrally run monopoly. It is time to let go.'[331]

> The NHS must become a values-based system where different health-care providers – in the public, private and voluntary sectors – provide comprehensive services to NHS patients within a common ethos; care free at the point of use, based on patient need and their informed choice and not their ability to pay. Who provides the service becomes less important than the service that is provided within a framework of clear national standards.[331]

Milburn predicted that this policy would be unpopular in some quarters, and he was right. The trade unions were furious and the BMA was predictably against the idea. Their concerns were increased further by reports in February that Milburn had up his sleeve a radical plan to use the private sector to the full, and to water down the historical commitment to comprehensive care. NHS service could be provided by the private sector under franchise deals.[332] Not surprisingly, some commentators thought Milburn was taking the NHS beyond Thatcherism. He even received what must have been an unwelcome commendation from Alain Enthoven for moving beyond the timid Thatcher reforms to a bold wide-open market.[333]

For the Department of Health the task of managing the NHS became one of overseeing a system, rather than of managing a single organisation. In its new role it was limited to four essential functions:

1 setting strategic direction by distributing resources and determining standards, and in particular moving policy towards a more explicit focus on improvements in public health
2 ensuring the integrity of the whole system by, for example, securing integrated information systems, staff training and development
3 developing the values of the NHS through education, training and policy development
4 securing accountability for funding and performance, including reports to Parliament.[306]

The NHS was to be encouraged to speak more for itself. The NHS Confederation was told that it should adopt a role independent of government.[322] In July 2001, at the Confederation Conference, the Department had drawn it into pay bargaining and gave it the lead in discussions about a new general practitioner contract. The new and independent Commission for Health Improvement would report on performance. A new cluster of bodies and organisations began to appear on the scene outside the Department of Health, but with a national role.

Franchising

Ministers thought that the management of NHS services could be invigorated, for a short time at least, by the introduction of internal and external franchising. Poorly performing trusts and health authorities would have their management team replaced by one from more successful organisations. There was an open national competition for the short list of managers who were judged capable of running a strategic health authority. The successful candidates were then invited to bid for a time-limited franchise. Nigel Crisp, the Permanent Secretary and Chief Executive, was directly involved in the whole process. The most senior civil servant in the Department was very much in charge of the most senior NHS appointments. Despite its commercial language the franchising process felt, at least to some of the participants, like an enhanced public service interview process of the kind used before in the NHS in the run-up to the 1974 and later reorganisations. Successful nationally short-listed candidates were then matched to authorities with the approval of local chairmen. The one substantial variation from the past was the ability of a chief executive to bring his or her own team with them. Franchising the management of failing trusts followed a similar path to internal transfers of management teams within the NHS in the early days, with a commercial franchise only coming along later. But even here the commercial companies recruited former NHS managers to lead their teams. New NHS services such as a network of diagnostic and treatment centres were to be built and perhaps managed by the private sector, preferably employing doctors and nurses from overseas. By the autumn of 2004, Labour was pushing for at least 15% of all NHS non-emergency surgery to be outsourced to the private sector. This was enough, they judged, to break the consultants' traditional cartel. The notion of public commissioning and private providing was gaining ground quickly, and was fuelled by new models of public interest companies epitomised by foundation status. Labour had, they thought, found the middle ground between 'state-run public' and 'shareholder-led private' structures. The Blair Government wanted 'no longer to run a nationalised industry but instead to oversee a system of care.'[306]

A historic investment decision

The biggest decisions of all for the Blair Government had always been focused on the funding questions. In April 2002, Blair and Brown, the Chancellor of the Exchequer, made what was an historic commitment to provide through general taxation, and an increase in National Insurance contributions, enough investment to get the NHS up to 9.4% of GDP by 2008. At this level England would, they claimed, be on a par with European levels of expenditure. However, with this new money had to come a faster rate of reform. The strategy unit in the Department of Health, which reported directly to ministers, burnt the midnight oil with Simon Stephens, who had by now moved to Downing Street as Health Policy Adviser, in shaping up the new reform programme. The Prime Minister and Alan Milburn were heavily involved, and Gordon Brown took a keen interest. The result was *Delivering the NHS Plan: next steps*,[334] which was announced to the NHS under the personal stamp of the Prime Minister,[335] and was modernised as the new cash began to flow into the system.

Planned NHS spending in the UK[363]

	£ billion
2002–03	65.4
2003–04	72.1
2004–05	79.3
2005–06	87.2
2006–07	95.9
2007–08	105.6

'The 1948 model was,' they claimed, 'simply inadequate for their needs.'[334] There were to be 15 000 more doctors, 30 000 more therapists and scientists, and 35 000 more nurses, midwives and health visitors. Sceptics wondered where these staff would come from, but professional training programmes began to expand and England started to plug the medium-term gap by recruiting from overseas, much to the discomfort of some European partners, who preferred to take English patients. In the new world, hospitals would be paid by results using a national tariff within a system that by 2004–05 was to be completely cash limited at the centre.[363] There would no longer be any national open-ended budgets. Patients would be allowed to choose the hospital at which they would be treated. Waiting lists for operations were planned to fall to a maximum of three months by 2008. Foundation hospitals, supposedly the best in the country, would occupy new territory as independent public benefit corporations able to settle their own pay and borrow capital from the markets. The NHS would have its own in-house bank. Blair had begun to adopt what looked very much like Thatcher-style solutions.

Foundation hospitals

Ideas about foundation status were, at first at least, very attractive to ambitious trust managers because of the promised escape from detailed central oversight and the ability to raise commercial capital for new development. However, the Treasury soon intervened and cooled everything down. 'Who underwrote these debts which had to remain on the public sector balance sheet?' they asked. There had to be limits and controls. The row was represented in the media as a fight between Milburn and Brown, and finally the Prime Minister had to get involved.[336] The Treasury stood its ground for a while, but eventually a compromise was struck which gave foundation hospitals a degree of limited control over capital expenditure, but within the overall expenditure envelope for the NHS. Foundation hospitals would not be allowed to fund their borrowing by a major expansion of private work, when the priority was to increase public-sector capacity.[336] Ardour cooled even more when it became clear that the idea had moved on from rewarding good performers with freedoms to substituting a slackening of central control for tighter local political control. Trust chairmen and non-executives began to worry that they might be disposed of if they had to go through a local election process. For some it was a case of out of the frying pan into the fire.

The trade unions were opposed from the start and some members, like Dave Prentis, the General Secretary of UNISON, forecast 'the end of healthcare as we know it' if the policy was pursued.[337] It was to take the Government until the end of 2003 to get foundation hospitals on to the statute book.

The underlying philosophy now was to be local empowerment and decentralisation within a national framework of standards and regulation. Increasing day-to-day control by Whitehall would end. Inspection and audit would be independent of the Department of Health. For how long would this last, the experienced observers wondered? There was also to be a rapprochement with the private sector. The management practices and structure of Kaiser Permanente, a prominent health insurer and provider in the USA, began to be quoted with enthusiasm. Americans began to be appointed to a few key posts in England.

Despite the fine words about devolution, the lines of accountability still ran directly to the door of the Secretary of State, who continued to chair the Modernisation Board. He was still very much in charge. National targets and national service frameworks still dominated local spending plans. The performance management processes were as bureaucratic and oppressive as ever, and had a new energy from the Downing Street Delivery Unit, which Blair had established immediately after the election under Lord Macdonald. This unit began to relate directly to parts of the NHS that were in trouble. The Department of Health itself was by now locked into a Whitehall service delivery process in which the Prime Minister took a close interest. Ministers were still up to their shoulders in details of operational management – everything from food to pay. The rhetoric and the reality were still far apart.

Dissonance

There was also a major dissonance in the system itself. Ministers kept explaining that their investment was paying off. A million more patients were being admitted for surgery than had been the case in 1997. Waiting times were lower. The number of general and acute beds had increased. Death rates from cancer and heart disease were sharply reduced.[338] The words were one thing, but the day-to-day experience was another. PCTs that took up over 50% of the NHS budget in April 2002, as health authorities and regional offices disappeared, expressed strong concern that they would inherit debts of £1.5 billion which would stifle them at birth.[339] Extra money poured into the NHS at the top but never seemed to arrive at the ward or surgery. It disappeared into pay rises for staff, overruns on drug prescribing in general practice and correcting long-standing underlying deficits. PCTs, which now had the lion's share of all the money, clamped down clinical expectations rather than encouraging them. There was a major row when the much-trumpeted new cancer money never arrived at the clinical coalface.[340] The House of Commons Select Committee on Science and Technology reckoned that half of the cash earmarked nationally for cancer had to be siphoned off to meet local deficits. Modernising the NHS was going to take a long time. If the centre had a core philosophy it kept changing. Suddenly patient choice jumped out of the Downing Street bag. Starting in London, every patient was to be given a choice of at least four hospitals in which to have their cold surgery. Competition within this sector of the NHS was suddenly legitimate. The embers of competition between hospitals began to glow again. To those in the field it had the whiff of illusions of the kind they had grown used to in a politically led NHS. Some managers in the field, and their boards, seriously believed that if they could hold on long enough it would be possible to surf their way to the next reorganisation. They did not need a change of government; just a cabinet reshuffle. Meanwhile the Conservatives started to talk about a system based on compulsory health insurance rather than general taxation.[341]

Localism

By now events were moving quickly. In February 2003, Milburn continued his process of redefining the NHS with a speech entitled 'Localism: from rhetoric to reality.'[338] Localism was the new political keyword. Milburn acknowledged that in its first term Labour had tried to change the NHS 'from the top down through a plethora of service targets, inspection regimes and national standards.' He said that 'it was now wrong to try to run the NHS nationally.' He was unrepentant about national targets, arguing that all large organisations have them: 'this absurd debate we have about targets versus autonomy is in my view the worst kind of philosophical reductionism. What you have to do is get the calibration right.'[255]

This meant, he said, placing limits on the role of Whitehall. The Government had to do less and the NHS had to do more. Accountability had to shift outwards to the communities they served, not upwards to the Department of Health.

Decentralisation within a framework of national standards was to be the new philosophy. It would lead, according to Nigel Crisp, to a reduction of about one-third of the Department of Health as they concentrated on 'steering, not rowing' the health and social care system.[342] Some, like Professor Roger Dyson, regarded this policy as a means of escaping from difficult national decisions in fields such as professional manpower which was now, in his view at least, an unholy mess.[343] Few regarded the downsizing as anything other than a short-term measure, and many doubted that it would actually be implemented. It did not feel short-term to all those civil servants in London and Leeds whose jobs and careers were suddenly at risk. Morale at the centre dropped like a stone.

The 14 directorates were replaced by three business groups. The membership of the Board on inception was as follows:

Department of Health, Management Board, July 2003[344,345]

Chief Executive/Permanent Secretary   Sir Nigel Crisp

Chief Medical Officer/Health and Social Care
Group Director   Sir Liam Donaldson
Oversees quality, health promotion, protection of the population and patient safety

Health and Social Care Delivery Group Director	Alan Bacon
Covers the performance of health and social care, the access programme, capacity programme workforce and IT	
Strategy and Business Development Group Director	Hugh Taylor
Covers communications, user experience and involvement and corporate work, including private offices	
Director of Policy	Andy McKeon
Director of User Experience and Chief Nursing Officer	Sara Mullally
Director of Communications	Sian Jarvis
Director of Finance and Investment	Richard Douglas

If one ignores the new Labour titles, this Board is not very far removed from all of its predecessors. Like them it had no formal status and operated under a cloak of confidentiality. Reporting to it was another Board called the Health and Social Care Delivery Board that had a membership which included all of the above plus the heads of separate businesses such as IT, access, research and development and human resources. Inside the Department the Strategy Unit, led by Chris Ham, continued to report directly to ministers.

The interface with the NHS was managed by means of a 'Top Team' which some saw as a replacement for the NHS Executive. This team included all of the Department of Health Directors, the National Clinical Directors and all of the SHA chief executives. Within the Department, 'executive'-type business was being consolidated under the control of John Bacon, who acted as Crisp's effective deputy.

The NHS together with its headquarters continued its everlasting change programme, and on 12 June 2003 it was given yet another Secretary of State, Dr John Reid, to provide leadership. He lasted less than two years.

Reid immediately softened Milburn's hard-line approach over the consultants' contracts and set out on a tour of the country to explain why patient choice was now top of the agenda. He also sought to breathe some new life into the public health debate after a third report by Derek Wanless (this time into public health),[346] with an extensive public consultation about how far governments should go in policy areas such as smoking and obesity. His role, he explained, 'was to lead not manage the NHS.' A straight answer to the question that Griffiths had suggested Florence Nightingale would have asked about the modern NHS, namely 'Who is in charge?', was still evaded.

Dr John Reid, Secretary of State

John Reid was born in 1947 in Scotland and educated in Coatbridge and Stirling University, where he read history and took a doctorate in Economic History. He has been MP for Motherwell since 1987 and has held positions as Minister of State for Defence 1997–98, Minister of Transport 1998–99, Secretary of State for Scotland May 1999–Jan 2000, and Secretary of State for Ireland Jan 2000–Oct 2002. He was Labour Party Chairman Oct 2002–

April 2003. He became Secretary of State for Health on 12 June 2003. After the general election in 2005 he moved to Defence.

Chapter 7

Reflections

Ever since the NHS was created, governments have struggled to manage it. By the mid-1980s ministers had injected general management into the system and created an NHS Chief Executive post located within the Department of Health. In England all the holders of this post came from an industry or NHS background. Only in Wales and Northern Ireland, where similar structures were in place, were chief executive appointments sometimes made from the ranks of the main Civil Service. In England, the NHS Chief Executive was accorded the rank of second Permanent Secretary, until Crisp became the first Permanent Secretary where the posts of Chief Executive and Permanent Secretary were combined.

Throughout this period politicians constantly wrestled with the tension between a national service and local decision making. For some, like Sir Chris France, a former Permanent Secretary, this was always the key question. Labour made postcode prescribing a big election issue, but eventually found themselves embracing postcode service provision (albeit within a tighter national framework) by moving to a primary care-led NHS. Local decision making creates variation in what is a nationally provided service.

Organisational change was a constant feature of every new plan for the NHS between 1974 and the present day. Nothing seemed to work for long. Those who expressed doubts or concerns about the wisdom of organisational change rarely won the argument. Ministers who declared themselves opposed to organisational change when they came into office soon found themselves promoting change on the grounds that it was a vital component of NHS improvement plans. Organisational change they could understand – it could be presented as progress and cost free. One of the consequences was a steady loss of experienced managers as they chose the early-retirement options that became available. The administrators of old, who had largely made up Roy Griffith's first crop of managers, were no longer coming up the system in sufficient numbers. Nurses, with their low professional salary ceilings, began to swell the ranks of middle and senior management, which was much better paid, particularly in fields such as mental health. Doctors moved into management positions in much smaller numbers. Ministers progressively stripped out various regional and intermediate tiers between the centre and the field either, on the grounds that they either impeded national policies or were simply unnecessary. Alan Milburn built up the national structures whilst his successor John Reid brought them down. Reducing management costs was always an attractive political option. Since the mid-1980s the regional or intermediate tiers between Whitehall and field authorities had been the focus for argument and change. They could be a very strong firebreak for ministers when things went wrong, and with the right leadership they could be a very effective means of ensuring that national targets were delivered on the ground. This was why Labour, having eradicated the last vestiges of the old regional health authorities, created strategic health authorities.

Each Secretary of State came to the health portfolio with an individual style and very mixed experience. Most either wanted to be hands on, or felt that they had no choice in the matter. They had to respond to every criticism or challenge that appeared in the media, even when it centred upon an individual or patient. Their political future depended on how they handled the problems that health always produced. The health policy agenda, from cancer to information technology to hospital food, was divided up between the members of a large ministerial team, all of whom wanted part of the action and a share of the headlines. Thus the NHS swung from detailed control from the centre to overt devolution, sometimes under the same Secretary of State when they were at different points on his or her personal learning curve. All saw themselves as executive chairmen, but some did try hard to create some distance from day-to-day operations. Bottomley in particular was happy to allow the NHS Executive to develop its own identity and even disagree with her, but like all her colleagues she kept a firm grip on the ultimate levers of power.

All attempts to separate policy from implementation and day-to-day management failed. In health the two are inextricably linked, except at the very highest levels of public policy which impact across the whole of the public sector. The constant battle to reduce the number of national targets was never won. Neither was the battle to keep a consistent policy line and the associated investment intact over an extended period of years. Priorities kept shifting and, as they did so, reporting systems became corrupted and tunes began to be played with the numbers. Today's priority was always more important than yesterday's. In their early years new leaders relied on a myriad targets until they realised that this did not work. The targets had, according to the Treasury, 'weighed down local managers and frontline staff with bureaucracy, distracted attention from key priorities, and hampered the ability of schools, hospitals and the police to deliver.'[371]

The best NHS managers, as judged by the centre, were those skilled at handling the policy ambiguities and the challenge of living with politicians. Health boards often found themselves trying to cope with mounting debt, which they were sometimes told to clear quickly and at other times instructed to manage via extended and often hopelessly optimistic recovery plans. Whatever their debts, they still had to deliver national targets in sensitive areas such as waiting-list management. The best strategic solutions were uncontroversial. Politically unpopular solutions, particularly those involving bed closures and shifts in service, were extremely difficult to get approved and were often vetoed by ministers if the issue rose to their level for resolution. The NHS Executive frequently found itself trying to broker difficult operational choices with ministers who were wary of political noise. With the demise of Community Health Councils, local authorities were given oversight authority to call controversial health plans in for local debate and, if they thought it appropriate, to refer them to a national NHS body for a second opinion. Local government was on the whole too preoccupied with its own problems to take this oversight role seriously.

The extra money that became available to the NHS with the NHS Plan went towards promoting nationally earmarked targets. There was little room for local discretion. However, by 2003–04 the sheer weight of the new investment was undoubtedly beginning to show results, but the dust of the political preparations for the new election masked them. Once more the NHS was going to get a good kicking with the emphasis this time on hospital cleanliness and access times to general practice.

The harsh truth is that politicians have neither the temperament nor the discipline for the long hard slog of policy implementation and the grind of day-to-day management. The political process and the media always have priority. A call from Parliament or the media always overrode a long planned visit to see local health services. Political careers are built on headline-breaking innovation and dramatic progress. The Civil Service, into which the chief executive and his team had to fit, proved to be a poor vehicle for managing a complex public service like health. It was designed for policy, not for operations.

Parliamentary accountability

Politicians of all parties have for many years felt that they had little choice but to run the NHS, and in this they were bolstered by what they were advised was a constitutional principle of some considerable importance. It was the principle of parliamentary accountability. This is centuries old and has played a central role in shaping the management of the NHS from its earliest days.

Under this doctrine ministers have to be accountable to Parliament for the manner in which public money is spent. Only they can stand at the dispatch box and explain their policies and defend their actions. Bevan, of course, took the concept well beyond cash with his statement that 'every time a maid kicks over a bucket of slops in a ward an agonised wail will go through Whitehall.'[35]

It was this doctrine that dominated the thinking of Stowe and his successors as they wrestled with the problems of introducing general management into an NHS that was growing in size and complexity with each passing year. The Griffiths Report and its powerful headline about Florence Nightingale searching for the person in charge had struck a cardinal point in the British constitutional process. However, the concept of parliamentary accountability is, as the Royal Commission of 1979 pointed out, a constitutional illusion. It is a myth.[16]

The idea that ministers could be omnipotent beings who know everything about the operation of their departments is clearly nonsense. David Hinchliffe MP, the Chairman of the Health Select Committee, put it as follows:

> It really is a nonsense to have this great kind of vision of parliamentary accountability which means that once in every five weeks I can ask one question of the Secretary of State if I am lucky. I think the idea of parliamentary accountability in health is largely mythical.[347]

Mythical it may be, but many parliamentarians would still be loath to give up even the smallest opportunity to hold government and its ministers to account. In recent years, health has always been the public service that puts government on the defensive as they strive to drive efficiency and limit the strain on the public purse. Even when they invest heavily, as Blair did, it still causes problems and is an easy target for opposition parties to attack.

Sir Robin Butler, the former head of the Civil Service, sought to distinguish between ministerial accountability and blame in the following terms: 'Ministers are accountable to Parliament for every last postage stamp, but not to blame if one is stuck upside down.'[348] In these terms the doctrine has been reworked so that ministers have to account for everything that happens in their department, but are not directly and personally accountable when things go wrong – a very convenient redefinition. One wonders what accountability really means when one observes that not a single health minister has ever resigned because of a failing in the NHS or, for that matter, following even the sternest criticism by a parliamentary committee. Bevan resigned on a matter of political principle, and Currie was sacked for a political gaffe and damage to the egg industry. Hunt resigned because of the war with Iraq. No minister resigned in the wake of the Bristol Inquiry, despite the fact that the problem centred on a nationally commissioned service, or for the failings at Ashworth Special Hospital in Liverpool, which was accountable directly to the Department of Health. Over the years, hundreds of NHS chairmen and managers have either resigned or been sacked. It seems that ministers are immune from everything except a judgement by their Prime Minister about their loyalty or competence. The issue of sacking a civil servant for an NHS failing never arises, even if they led in the policy area involved. An NHS chief executive on a five-year renewable contract may be more vulnerable, but even here, as the Fallon Report[210] concluded, the Chief Executive of the NHS is not in charge in the accepted sense of that expression. He is a civil servant and an adviser to the Secretary of State.

There was an illuminating row at the Home Office in 1995 on the question of the difference between political and operational authority for prisons. The Director of the Prison Service lost. Michael Howard, then Conservative Home Secretary, won. The power was his to take away as well as his to delegate. If he wanted to have the final say in prison regimes or management, he would have it.[349, 350]

Kenneth Clarke takes the view that parliamentary accountability is a concept nursed more by civil servants than by politicians:

> That's the Civil Service view. It defends their position, that's why civil servants have to know everything that you are doing, because their minister is accountable to Parliament. The civil servants are keener on that than ministers are – for a variety of reasons – some noble, some ignoble. Ministers are not too averse to getting rid of the responsibility for bedpans in Batley if they can.[38]

Within Parliament, oversight for health is focused primarily within two committees. These are the Health and Social Services Select Committee, which concentrates principally on policy and therefore usually calls ministers to give evidence, and the Public Accounts Committee, which reviews expenditure and efficiency and usually calls for evidence from the permanent secretary and other accounting officers.

The NHS chief executives and their senior colleagues spent a great deal of time preparing for and attending these committees, sometimes, as one senior parliamentarian put it, 'because ministers did not want to go.' Some of the hearings were overtly political, particularly during the period when Labour was in opposition. The first permanent secretary got called less and less often by the Public Accounts Committee. Nichol and Langlands (who were second permanent secretaries) both appeared more often than any other permanent secretary in Whitehall. Langlands went on 26 occasions.[216] The Public Accounts Committee wanted to see the man who was supposed to be in charge of the NHS, where most of their questions and challenges were focused. The briefings, which produced huge volumes of paper, went on for weeks before the hearings themselves, which lasted for only a few hours.

The committees rarely distinguished between political and managerial questioning when dealing with the NHS chief executive. Many of the hearings were brutal and partisan. So much for the neutral civil servant unless, in the eyes of Parliament at least, these particular civil servants were regarded as being somehow different from their colleagues – public service managers rather than mandarins in the classic mode. Appearing before Parliament represented a major time commitment for both Nichol and Langlands that might have been better spent running the NHS.

So why does every health authority and its chairman have to be accountable directly to the Secretary of State? Why is hierarchy such a troublesome concept? Why in the days of Paige could the regional chairmen not report to him as Chairman of the National Management Board? Was it because such a change would have caused tension with regional chairmen or was there really an important constitutional principle at stake? Were regional chairmen being seen as political advisers and thus entitled to sit in the kitchen cabinet? Why did Alan Langlands have to admit at a public inquiry that he did not manage the NHS but only the NHS Executive, despite the fine words in the formal statement of accountabilities about his responsibility for the management and performance of the NHS in England? The public thought that he managed the NHS, as did many staff in the NHS. It suited Whitehall to sustain the illusion. Nigel Crisp, the holder of the combined post of chief executive and permanent secretary, is still described as being directly accountable to the Secretary of State for the management and performance of the NHS in England.[334] One wonders if he will use the 'Langlands defence' when his turn comes to face an inquiry, or whether he will be the first Permanent Secretary to resign on the grounds of a service failure for which some think that he is ultimately accountable.

In any case, if the principle is so important, how is it that John Reid could decide (without a major row) that foundation hospitals would not be accountable to him? Parliament would have to address their questions to the trust chair.[377]

Public or private

Only recently, under Blair, Milburn and Reid, has the notion of overseeing a system rather than managing a service been seriously aired. In the modern world, public ownership might now mean public commissioning and standard setting, not necessarily public management. Foundation trusts will escape the direct control of the Secretary of State and will instead be accountable to an independent regulator, who is in turn accountable to Parliament. Foundation trust chief executives will have no formal relationship with the Chief Executive of the NHS. Private hospitals are now legitimate providers of NHS care. Primary care might even be run by private companies.[369] Hospital consultants go a step further, arguing that a publicly funded NHS will never work.[370] A pluralistic NHS is still a challenging political concept for some, particularly for the trade unions.

Politicians were elected to guide and lead our society and to shape our values and priorities. The big questions about what kind of health delivery system we should have are properly those for elected politicians. What they should not do is attempt to run complex services like the NHS on a day-to-day basis. This is a task for which most do not have the necessary instinct, skills or training.

Civil Service culture and role

The parliamentary accountability concept is complicated by another perhaps equally important concept, relating to the role and status of civil servants with its emphasis on utter impartiality, objective advice and public invisibility. If civil servants operated under their own name, under delegated powers in services as close to the public as the NHS, they would become accountable, visible and lose their impartiality. How could they explain and defend their actions in public, sometimes under pressure from the opposition parties, without being accused of being partisan? If civil servants believed with a passion in the policies that they were implementing we would be well on the way to a politicised Civil Service. They have to remain neutral. The next government might require them to undo everything they have done for its predecessor.

Passion is an emotion for ministers, not for civil servants. Everything that a civil servant does must be in the name of ministers. The implementation plans that they adopt are mechanised, well ordered and rational, but they lack a driving personal commitment by those in charge. Those who want others to change must have a belief in their own arguments. Explaining what ministers want has nothing like the same impact. This is part of the reason why the Civil Service has been so poor at policy implementation and why ministers get so frustrated and want to become directly and personally involved.

It was partly to ease this problem that Next Steps Agencies were created from 1988 onwards. They were designed to manage those parts of the government machine that handled routine business in organisations that could operate with a modicum of operational independence within a clear ministerial policy framework. The Passport Office and the Benefits Office are among those best known to the public, but there are now many others. Each has its own chief executive with accounting officer status, and all employ civil servants. Although they are free of ministerial involvement in day-to-day matters, they still remain technically accountable to ministers. Thus, as the Government explained to a Select Committee, 'setting up agencies within departments will not result in changes to the existing constitutional arrangements.' They were seen as organisations undertaking routine and well-defined tasks, not as policy makers. The civil servants they employed were to be specifically trained for the work they would do, rather than general policy. For a while it was planned to move the Modernisation Agency to Next Steps status, but eventually ministers decided that this model was not suitable for an agency whose role was continual improvement. The application for agency status was withdrawn in December 2003.[351]

Next Step Agencies do from time to time have difficulty with their head-quarters, which set their terms of reference and service standards and are usually keen to stress the notion of one department. Turf fights are common, particularly when the agency runs into operational problems when implementing changes of policy. The Department of Health played the same controlling game with the NHS

Executive in its insistence on recognising the importance of the wider Department of Health of which the Executive was but a part.

However, what is surprising is the rigidity with which the policy of ministerial accountability was applied within the Department of Health. With the creation of an Executive one might have expected to see some explicit delegation by the Secretary of State of operational authority of the kind commonly found in large organisations in both the public and private sectors. The scheme of delegation would set out in some detail the extent to which authority had been delegated by ministers (usually within financial or other limits), as well as making it clear which decisions were not delegated and thereby reserved for ministers. It could have been done without breaching any constitutional principles. The minister would remain ultimately accountable. However, it would have resulted in civil servants exercising executive power in a very explicit manner. This was not how the Civil Service managed its relationship with ministers, and a new Health Executive was not sufficient reason to change a well-established pattern of working. The NHS Executive had to fit in and remember that it was part of the Civil Service. Meetings of the Executive were not open to the public, and attendance by outsiders was strictly limited. The circulation of minutes was strictly controlled, and they were labelled as strictly confidential. The word 'decide' had been banned from the early days.

It might be argued that the health version of Next Steps was the creation of special health authorities such as NICE, the Prescription Pricing Authority, NHS Estates or, more recently, NHS Direct. However, these have a statutory basis and are rather different. For example, they do not insist that all their employees are civil servants. Some hold their Board meetings in public. For the NHS Executive to have operated in such a manner they would have needed a clear statutory or Next Steps base from which to operate, and this was a step too far for both Whitehall and ministers. However, foundation trusts do represent a radical break with history. They will have to be controlled via national quality standards and primary care trust commissioners. The next time there are questions in Parliament about bodies being stored in chapels rather than the mortuary, the Secretary of State will be able to refer the question to the foundation trust and perhaps their Regulator.

Despite the fact that the various Executives remained firmly within the fold of the wider Department of Health and acted as advisers to ministers, they were able in a number of areas, such as information technology, to develop new policy and get on with its implementation with only a token involvement by ministers. However, the vast majority of the policy shifts were conceived and initiated by ministers, including many in service areas such as maternal care, mental health and the role of hospitals. Some were no doubt prompted or seeded by the Executive, but most appear not to have been. Ministers retained their list of personal policy areas covering everything from revenue allocations to security regulations in mental health and food in hospitals, and ministers' private offices made sure that no one forgot them. Ministers who were slow to make decisions in unfamiliar territory were a real problem. In non-political areas most ministers simply accepted the advice given to them by officials. It was not a very effective way to manage one of the largest organisations in the economy.

Under the Labour Government the role of the political adviser grew significantly, as did that of the Director of Strategy. They operated alongside but outside the formal machinery, and had a substantial influence over both general policy and communication strategies. They watched the media and opinions in their focus groups very carefully indeed and maintained a close link with the policy advisers in Downing Street. The Downing Street advisers played a significant role in shaping health policy.

In one respect the top team at the Department of Health did change under Crisp. By 2004 he was able to argue that his Department Board consisted of two traditional civil servants, two recruited from the private sector, two NHS managers and two clinicians. It was, he claimed, an unusual board for Whitehall, and of the top 70 civil servants in his department, 20 were clinicians.[372] By 2005, Crisp was advertising for external non-executives to serve on his Board.

The various NHS Executives had no corporate status or standing orders. There was no question of members taking votes. Despite this, a number of attempts were made to develop a distinctive identity, as if it did exercise an independent function. For a while it produced an annual report and a house magazine, and had a separate web page. It had its own communication team focused primarily on internal communication to the NHS. The move to Leeds was designed in part to give the Executive space, but it did not work. Ken Jarrold explained that it did not work 'because the DoH is part of an immensely strong civil service culture which, like the human body, will reject external transplants.' There was a lot of organ rejection going on in the Department of Health.[218] The power remained with ministers in London and their civil servants.

The NHS Executive within the Department of Health was a corporate illusion from beginning to end. The quality of the Chief Executives gave it an authority beyond its formal status in the organisation, but it would have been better titled an Advisory Board, for that was what it was. In this respect Victor Paige got it right from the start.

The chief executives

The first two chief executives, Paige and Peach, came from industry. The next two, Nichol and Langlands, came from within the NHS. All of them carried a senior Civil Service rank on appointment (second Permanent Secretary), but the first three came into the Department of Health on a seconded basis. This avoided both a difficult negotiation about remuneration with the individual selected and the creation of troublesome precedents within the Civil Service. Langlands was the first chief executive to be appointed on a substantive Civil Service grade. Conveniently, this was at a time when senior Civil Service posts were being re-evaluated. The NHS chief executive post scored very well indeed, so the assimilation was easy. Every chief executive was appointed on a short-term renewable contract, the decision about renewal being in the hands of the Prime Minister. If nothing else did, this marked out these permanent secretaries as different from the rest of the Civil Service community. Crisp, who also came from the NHS, was the first to be appointed to the combined post of chief executive and first permanent secretary.

With the exception of Paige, the chief executives were recruited in accordance with Civil Service rules and procedures. Ministers were not directly involved in the appointments although, as with all Civil Service appointments at this level, the Prime Minister's approval was required. Virginia Bottomley has since made it plain that ministers would claim a right to veto the appointment of a candidate with whom they felt they could not work. In any case it was simply inconceivable that the chief executive of the NHS could be appointed without prior consultation with the Secretary of State. This was not a classic Civil Service shuffle and promotion process – it was assumed in advance that the successful candidate would most probably come from outside the ranks of the established Civil Service. This situation will no doubt change now that the posts of chief executive and permanent secretary have been combined although Crisp, a man from the NHS, felt sufficiently confident of his combined role to throw his hat in the ring for the job as Cabinet Secretary in 2005.

The appointments were made on the basis of experience, intellect and the ability to operate within a team. The successful candidate had to be able to accept political leadership and use influence and persuasion as their principal tools. An individual with strong personal ideas would be dangerous, as would one who demanded personal powers and authority. The successful candidate had to possess a finely tuned political antenna and learn the subtle art of living with politicians and adjusting to their moods and ideas.

This was not the profile that Mrs Thatcher had in mind when the first Management Board was created. She wanted an experienced leader with energy, ideas and a public persona of their own. She positively did not want a civil servant in the job. She misjudged the attitudes of both her ministers and the Civil Service. Ministers like the power that comes with running a large Department of State. In a moment of typical candour, Kenneth Clarke explains that he was rather annoyed when Roy Griffiths was first foisted upon him by Downing Street: 'I was just beginning to have ideas, as all young ministers do, and planned to put the world of the NHS to rights.'[38] He wanted to make his own policy and draw on his own ideas rather than have it done for him by a businessman whom he hardly knew. Alan Milburn made a similar point from a different perspective when he said that 'central bureaucracies create work. Politicians, for good reasons, not bad, want to get their hands dirty. We want to pull levers that make changes happen.'[255] In 2003, the Department of Health had five ministers, all of whom wanted to get their hands dirty. It was far too many.

Relationships at the top

Relationships at the top of all organisations are inevitably complex, and this is particularly true when leadership is diffused. The roles of the permanent secretary, chief executive and Chief Medical Officer contained a significant degree of overlap of both interest and authority. Each had to be careful when managing their relationship with the others. It is a great credit to all those involved that, despite occasional turf battles waged by their subordinates, the relationship between the principals never appears to have seriously broken down. The permanent secretary was always first among equals, but as the big battalions of staff moved to the Executive that role began to diminish, and eventually of course the two were rolled into one. Whether a single person can ever be a big hitter both in the NHS and in Whitehall remains to be seen. If, as planned, the Department does indeed distance itself from operational matters in the NHS,

Crisp's replacement will probably be a career civil servant and the chief executive part of the job might be discarded. We will have turned full circle.

The relationship between the Chief Medical Officer and the chief executive seems to have varied over time. However, as the Department became more closely involved with clinical practice via national service frameworks and the like, the CMOs took their seat on the Executive much more seriously, and rather than delegating this role to a subordinate, joined the Executive team themselves. The Chief Nursing Officer had joined the Executive almost from the start, and over time collected responsibility for broader policy areas such as quality and mental health.

Politicians have related to the top management of the NHS in different ways. Conservative ministers liked to operate through the chairmen of regional health authorities. With some Tory ministers they were able to join the kitchen cabinet. They were expected to be loyal supporters of Government policies and act rather like political advisers on mood and opinion within the NHS. Bottomley even kept them on as what she called her 'Lord Lieutenants' in the field long after their Boards had disappeared. Labour ministers chose another path. They largely ignored the chairmen (now appointed by an independent commission) and related instead down the chief executive network.

Under the Labour Government the role of political adviser grew, adding yet another complication to the top of the office.

An independent NHS corporation

The idea of an independent corporation to run the NHS has been around for some years. A BMA review of the future of the NHS in 1967 mooted the idea, but dismissed it in the same short paragraph as it also dismissed the idea of a national sweepstake. The Fulton Committee in 1968 had suggested the hiving off of activities, including those in social fields, to autonomous public bodies. The Royal Commission on the NHS considered such an idea but thought that there was more to be gained at that time from making improvements within the existing statutory framework. Norman Fowler, in his memoirs entitled *Ministers Decide*, commented:

> By the end of my stay in health, I had become convinced that it would be possible to create a health commission with its own chief executive or chairman. Nothing will now take health out of politics, but a commission could produce a more efficient service. The advantage would be that ministers and civil servants would not be involved in day-to-day management.[84]

The Thatcher review considered an independent corporation, but eventually rejected the idea, as did Virginia Bottomley during her term in office. All it would do, she decided, would be to create another organisation to join the chorus of those demanding more money from government. Every problem would be linked back to resources and end up back on her desk, but without the detailed powers to sort out priorities. In any case her advisers would have explained to her that she was already reorganising the Department on the basis that it was almost impossible to disentangle policy and implementation. You could not put the whole Department of State into a corporation – the Treasury would never have stood for it.

As France puts it, 'the NHS was never an industry to be managed by an Independent Board. It is a branch of the body politic and will be for as long as it is publicly funded.'[120]

It took another government and a different industry to demonstrate that it was possible to take both operations and strategy out of Whitehall. The Strategic Railway Authority handles railway industry policy and acts as the commissioner of services – or it did until 2004, when Whitehall pulled some of these powers back and announced that the Rail Authority would be wound up. This way forward was not a million miles away from the English Health Authority idea first set out for Norman Fowler by Ken Stowe in 1985. This move did of course require primary legislation, an option that was not available to Stowe, and this was why an alternative path had to be chosen.

To take the analogy further, privately operated trains run on Railtrack's publicly owned system just as private or independent providers could provide services to a publicly funded and commissioned NHS.

However, there are other powerful arguments for wanting a higher degree of separation between politicians and the day-to-day management of the NHS. As things stand at present, the opposition parties are bound constantly to challenge the Government about their competence in managing the NHS. It is an easy target. It is such a huge organisation and medicine is still such an inexact science that something is always bound to go awry. Everything from poor communications between doctors and patients to difficulties in responding to surges in medical emergencies can be blamed on the politicians who have put themselves in charge. Attacks on NHS bureaucracy are legitimate for all parties, whether in government or not.

In the run-up to an election (now counted in half-years rather than weeks) the abuse gets more intense and any decisions with even an edge of controversy are shelved. The NHS is not allowed to defend itself during the political war games that take place immediately prior to an election. Like the rest of the public services, it has to go into purdah until it is all over. However, things got much tougher than usual in the period when Labour was in opposition, for they made it plain that many managers would be sacked if they won the election. There would be a price to be paid by those who had introduced the Conservative internal market reforms with too much enthusiasm. Local MPs individually threatened some managers. Nichol and Langlands worried about their future should the Government change, and so did some of their immediate colleagues with a health background. In their case a loss of position was the end of a career, not a move to another part of Whitehall. Although they were all civil servants, they expected to be treated differently.

There is also the largely unexplored question of how far the decision-making processes of the NHS are affected by improper political bias. Suspicions about the impartiality of the resource allocation process are deep-rooted, and decisions about controversial changes in marginal constituencies are sometimes very suspect. A review undertaken for the TV programme *Panorama* in 1997[352] demonstrated that a significant number of service changes had been blocked on what were judged locally to be party political grounds, principally that they could be presented as cuts by the opposition. The credit that Labour deserves for giving up patronage over paid non-executive appointments to health bodies, by creating an independent commission to fulfil this task and another to advise on controversial planning issues, has been diluted by their early penchant for double-counting new investment and feeding the media with a barrage of announcements about centrally targeted money, no matter how small the amounts.

NHS: national or local control

The balance between central strategic control and local discretion is always a problem in large organisations, whether they are in the public or the private sector. Throughout the 'executive years' the centralisation screw has been turning, and with good reason. A number of inquiries had highlighted poor performance, all of which had led to pressure for tighter national standards and service frameworks. Medicine itself and the technologies that supported it had demanded centralised investment and provision, as had the shifts in medical education and the associated reductions in doctors' hours of work. Hospitals began to merge and operate within networks of care, and general practitioners began to operate within larger partnerships. Information technology as applied in healthcare, which had been bogged down for years in a myriad local solutions, was slowly adjusting to a narrower range of options most evident in the field of general practice operating systems.

Clinical networks in fields such as cancer, which seek to fit together a complex set of services that are managed separately by different parts of the system, struggle with the tension between network and local ownership. With budgets locked in the individual hospitals, network-based decision making has been slow to develop. As a consequence, the majority of networks have remained collaborative rather than managed.

In a national service, local variation in service has always been a problem. By the late 1990s expenditure per head of population had been more or less evened out. However, at a time when resources were tight someone had to determine priorities. The political problems began when local health authorities started to make decisions about local entitlement to new drugs or services. It made sense, but the politics were a minefield. Conservative ministers did not want explicit lists of low-priority treatment areas to appear. Labour had made this a political issue in the run-up to the general election by campaigning against GP fundholding because, they claimed, it created a two-tier service and what they called postcode prescribing. It was a national not a local health service, they insisted. Whether one lived in Brighton or Gateshead was irrelevant – everyone was entitled to free comprehensive care. This led eventually to the notion of local control within a national framework of regulation and inspection. NICE would make national judgements about clinical effectiveness and particularly about drugs, and once ministers had accepted their recommendations everyone would apply them, thus reducing local variations. However, as the Labour Government is discovering, this is not easy to achieve and primary care trusts will resist more national targeting and demand more freedom to make local decisions that will once again produce variations in service at a local level. There was an enormous row towards the end of 2002 when Milburn discovered that his nationally earmarked money for mental health and cancer had been hijacked on the way by managers pursuing local priorities and other national objectives, such as financial balance. Plurality of provision will produce variations in service. It is variations in basic entitlement rather than variations in the quality of service provided that create difficulties of principle.

For decades now the health industry has been consolidating into larger units in order to conserve scarce specialist skills and achieve economies of scale. Despite this, the Labour Government decided in 2003 to block hospital rationalisation plans unless local communities agreed to them. Of course they rarely do. Single-issue politics, such as those demonstrated at Kidderminster where those fighting to save a local general hospital won both the parliamentary seat and took over control of the local council, can explain this policy shift far more than any rational health policy. One observer, Professor Roger Dyson, regards what he calls 'a surrender' to the status quo as 'an appalling abandonment of leadership, which they knew must have negative consequences for the public's health.' 'This was,' he claims, 'the point at which Labour lost the new NHS.'[343] It seems quite likely that the Labour Party, which is now promoting locality policies, is reorganising against the technological and economic grain.

As Rudolf Klein put it, 'the NHS has continued to march to the tune of changes in the technology of medicine and professional attitudes rather than ministerial bidding.'[117]

Leadership

The question 'Who leads the NHS?' has many answers. The NHS chief executive never became, or was never allowed to become, the kind of leader that Mrs Thatcher had in mind. She wanted someone to lead from the front and stamp his or her personality on the whole organisation. Langlands actually eschewed such leadership, arguing instead that the leader's role at the centre was in stimulating teamwork and in the creation of space for local leaders. It was, he argued, simply impracticable for one person to lead one of the largest organisations in Europe. He could lead a headquarters team and perhaps give leadership to NHS managers in the field, but not the whole of the NHS. Doctors, nurses and others would look for leadership to their local employers and the leaders of their professions or trade unions. Politicians have never led the NHS, and it is unlikely that they ever will. Far from leading the NHS, most end up fighting it.

The relationship between managers in the field and the chief executive was changed significantly when the Executive moved fully into the Civil Service. Suddenly the headquarters of the NHS was part of a different culture, with different loyalties and terms and conditions of service for staff. The Executive began to act more and more in Civil Service mode, with minutes of conversations being recorded and circulated widely, and option papers being sought prior to almost any decision. Decisions were rarely made on the spot – they had to be routed upwards to ministers via their red boxes. Decision making was slow. The NHS had its own bureaucratic traditions, of course, but they were less dependent on the written word and usually far more action oriented. There was now a constant concern about the media reaction to local decision making. Judgements about political reaction began to play a greater role in shaping change. The crucial importance of protecting ministers' backs was made plain to all and produced a sharp increase in the level of upward reporting. A good civil servant wanted to brief his or her minister before problems hit the press, not after the event. The problems that had previously been absorbed by the regional tier now went straight to the top. Ministers saw more, and because mainly problems were being reported upward, it was usually bad news.

Of all the Secretaries of State, Alan Milburn tried hardest to bring the health professions on board with his modernisation plans. He gave them seats on his Modernisation Board and drew them into thinking about the NHS plan. He created clinical 'czars' to bring leading national experts closer to the centre of power. It all had a positive short-term impact but did not last, for in truth the professions recognised that they were there to be persuaded that the latest Government idea was right, rather than being invited to join the inner circle of policy makers. It also quite quickly became clear to professional leaders how dangerous it was to be seen by their members as being too close to the political process. Professional self-interest is often a more powerful force than the greater good of the community or the NHS. On matters of pay and conditions of service Milburn was to find the BMA as difficult as his predecessor had. After delivering the biggest increase in investment in the history of the NHS, instead of being fêted like a hero by the NHS he found himself embattled in public rows about doctors' contracts.

Dr Ian Bogle, the GPs' leader and one of those admitted to the inner sanctum, was particularly critical of the Labour Government when he retired in the summer of 2003. He told the BMA conference, in what was described as a savage attack, that 'the fundamental NHS principle of care based on need has been superseded by care based on numbers.'[353]

He also attacked what he called 'corporate bullying by government which had left staff "in fear of their jobs and futures" if they failed to meet unrealistic targets.'[353]

The NHS has followed central policy leads throughout its history, but often with reluctance. The centre almost always blunted its own impact on the service with too many targets and a lack of consistency in seeing changes through to full implementation. Excellent policy initiatives such as Health of the Nation, which need sustaining over generations, slip away in the hurly-burly of day-to-day political life.[138, 354] Nichol and Langlands battled with ministers on this issue and although they sometimes won a respite, it was only ever temporary. The excitement at the centre is about new ideas that capture the headlines, not the long slog of implementation.

Chief executives and the media

All of the NHS chief executives were heavily restrained in their relationships with the media. They had to make sure that they did not tread on ministers' toes, or worse still steal their limelight. Nichol got into the most serious trouble within Whitehall by squashing a story that had been put out by Robin Cook, the then Labour health spokesman, that the Conservative Government was intent on privatising the NHS. 'It was simply not true,' he said, and for that he nearly lost his job. Opposition politicians were not best pleased by his intervention, which had been prompted by William Waldegrave, but his fellow mandarins were furious. This sounded like a political permanent secretary in action. The next thing would be short-term contracts for senior civil servants who changed with each government. Nichol, Langlands and Crisp did talk to the press, but largely behind the scenes, sharing background material with trusted journalists. They only appeared on television at times of minor crisis. Good news, new investment and really serious problems were news to be handled by ministers. All of the chief executives addressed professional conferences open to the press, but they were cautious and temperate in their language. They explained rather than evangelised about government thinking. They reserved their passion for private meetings with close and trusted colleagues.

Towards the end of his time as chief executive, Langlands did speak out publicly about the prospect of increased charges for patients. 'Bevan resigned,' he said, 'in his determination to stand by this principle. I think I would do the same.'[355] It was a clear shot across the bows of those policy advisers who were contemplating such a step. However, given the left-wing credentials of his Secretary of State, it was not an immediate problem, although it might have become one had the Government changed while he was still in office. It is inconceivable that Nigel Crisp could make such a statement in his combined role as permanent secretary and chief executive. However, he did stretch the boundaries somewhat in October 2003 when he wrote to *The Times* to correct a story about cuts in the number of hospital beds,[356] and in December 2003, when he presented a very upbeat report on progress in modernising the NHS. The politicians had calculated that he was more likely to be believed than they were.

Nichol and Langlands both faced the prospect of a change of Government within their term of office, and wondered about their prospects. Duncan Nichol would almost certainly have been replaced had Labour won the election. Langlands survived the transition successfully, but found it very uncomfortable, as he had believed in what he had been trying to achieve.

A tentative judgement

Few will challenge the huge benefits that this country has received from its core of incorruptible and neutral civil servants. However, in the last 30 years they have been asked to undertake an extended range of functions within a culture designed for policy advice. Some routine functions have performed well in Next Steps Agencies at a distance from day-to-day politics, but that step was never taken with the NHS. Instead, Whitehall tried to run the organisation from the centre with managers drafted in from the field. This never really worked. Managers running services like health cannot be invisible and impartial. To do their job well they need to believe in what they are doing with a passion and remain around long enough to deliver.

Alain Enthoven, who returned to the UK in 2001 to look again at the NHS, judged the Thatcher reforms to have failed because of poor implementation and too much political interference.[357]

Management of the NHS from the centre by politicians has not worked very well at all. It lacks a consistent core of values and direction, leadership is too diffused, and the system is reorganised too often in the name of progress.

Alternatives

At the start of 2003 the headquarters of the NHS were still firmly secured in Whitehall, close to the centre of government. However, the intention to go down the path of devolution had been signalled. There were discussions about the Modernisation Agency moving to Next Steps status (later aborted by ministers), but the national targets were still in place and continued to grow. Alan Milburn resigned in the summer of 2003 to spend more time with his family. The new Secretary of State, Dr John Reid, brought his own ideas and attitudes to the job. His early move was to announce his plan to lead rather than to manage the NHS. He told the Health Select Committee in October 2003 that 'politicians and civil servants should focus on strategic issues rather than the day-to-day management of the NHS.' He also announced swingeing cuts in the size of the Department of Health, from 3600 to 2200 within a year. Half of this number would actually disappear, but the balance would transfer to other national bodies. Once again the temptation to spin could not be resisted. Strategic health authorities, primary care trusts and the myriad *ad hoc* national bodies were warned that they, too, would be reviewed in order to see what cuts could be made.[358] The Tory opposition piled in behind them with promises of even greater cuts. As the election drew closer, John Reid and his team of ministers were pushed back to the operational detail. The Blair Government claims to have learned the hard way that they have been too keen to control schools, hospitals and the police from the centre through endless national targets and inspection systems. Localism is now the buzzword. Foundation hospital models are being refined and developed for schools and other parts of the public services. For some this is little more than a shift from national political control to local political control. For them it is out of the frying pan into the fire. In the longer term the Blair Government may well seek to get out of the provider side of health altogether, but the politics of doing so will be daunting.

At about the same time that Alan Milburn was acknowledging that the NHS could not be run from Whitehall, David Blunkett was making the same point about the Home Office and crime reduction, and receiving much flak for doing so. In an address to the Labour Party Spring Conference in 2002 he told delegates that there was a limit to the power of ministers to improve schools, hospitals and transport:

> Who to hold to account and for what is a key question we must address. At the moment we have the worst of all worlds. Ministers are presented as having responsibility for aspects of our life over which they do not have direct control. The Home Secretary is blamed for a rise in crime. Yet the police have operational independence. We need a public debate about where power lies in contemporary society. We cannot run or do everything in twenty-first century Britain.[359]

Blunkett got little sympathy from the media, who ran the story under the headline 'Don't blame us, guv.'[359] It is not yet clear how far and how fast the foundation movement will go, or whether it will indeed create any clear water between politicians and NHS providers. Speculation about the organisations that commission healthcare moving away from direct control by Whitehall was clearly part of Milburn's long-term strategy.

So is there a credible alternative way forward? Is an NHS corporation like the BBC simply impracticable? Is it time to create an English Health Authority to run the pluralistic system that together forms the NHS in England, or an NHS corporation as suggested by the King's Fund?[360] It would clearly operate to a contract agreed with the Department (perhaps now the Ministry) of Health, which would maintain accountability for the wider protection of the public health. The English Health Authority would operate in the middle ground created by Labour between the public and private sectors. Day-to-day management would be in the hands of a full-time executive team that would control the performance of the myriad public and private providers. Primary care trusts appointed by the English Health Authority could continue to provide a powerful local focus for commissioning within their national framework. A national hypothecated tax would simplify funding streams. As long as a capital debt could be serviced within approved revenue streams, the authority could have direct access to capital markets. Membership of the authority itself might include elected members from any new English regions as well as talented people from a wide spectrum of society, including patients and staff representatives. The Independent Appointments Commission would appoint members, but the Chairman would have to be someone in whom ministers had complete confidence. They would have to be involved in the chairman selection and renewal process.

Although the English Health Authority would be accountable to the Secretary of State, it could by convention be called to account directly by parliamentary committees. The staff of the English Health Authority could be civil servants specially trained and recruited for work in the health sector or, more likely, drawn from within the NHS. The public service manager model would be used rather than the Whitehall mandarin. The NHS could have a leader who lived and operated within the NHS culture. The accountability of the staff would be to their chief executive and his or her board.

Such an organisation might be better able to go with the grain of technology and science, adopt and hold to longer-term strategies and yet leave space for localism. This option leaves in place a small but still very important Department of Health with broad public health responsibilities and default powers in the event of system breakdown. Other countries have solved this problem by grouping health with other related policy areas, such as consumer affairs. In this way health retains a seat at the cabinet table.

Regional government might offer another way forward and provide an economic framework large enough to meet the demands of clinical science, but within a democratic framework. Local politicians are unlikely to be more competent than their national counterparts at day-to-day management, so the same arguments about segregation would have to apply.

John Reid edged closer to the separation point at the Labour Party Conference in October 2004 when he explained that his role would be limited to that of a custodian of the NHS and provider of finance as the devolution of the service continued.

The search for the best way to manage the provision of health services has to continue and keep up with developments in medicine. The Government needs to provide leadership in the field of health policy and withdraw from operational management. It will need a really strong politician to cover this transition and make it stick.

References

1 Ministerial Membership of DHSS 1970–88; www.psr.keele.ac.uk/table/york/dhss.html
2 Interview with Sir Kenneth Stowe, London, August 2001.
3 *A Chronology of State Medicine: public health, welfare and related services in Britain 1966–1999*; www.chronology.ndo.org.uk
4 DHSS (1968) *National Health Service: the administrative structure of the medical and related services in England.* HMSO, London.
5 Royal Commission on Local Government (1969) *Redcliffe Maud Report. Report of the Royal Commission on Local Government.* HMSO, London.
6 DHSS (1970) *National Health Service: the future structure of the National Health Service in England.* HMSO, London.
7 Central Health Services Council (1971) *Harvard Davies Report on the Organisation of GP Group Practice.* HMSO, London.
8 DHSS (1971) *Better Services for the Mentally Handicapped.* DHSS, London.
9 DHSS (1972) *Whittington Report. Report of the Committee of Inquiry into Whittington Hospital.* HMSO, London.
10 DHSS (1972) *National Health Service Reorganisation: England.* HMSO, London.
11 DHSS (1972) *Management Arrangements for the Reorganised National Health Service (the Grey Book).* HMSO, London.
12 DHSS (1973) *Collaboration with Local Government: report published from the Working Party on Collaboration between the NHS and Local Government on its activities to the end of 1972.* HMSO, London.
13 DHSS (1974) *Democracy in the National Health Service.* HMSO, London.
14 DHSS (1976) *Three Chairmens' Report. Regional Chairmens' Inquiry into the Working of the DHSS in Relation to Regional Health Authorities.* Department of Health and Social Security, London.
15 DHSS (1976) *Resource Allocation Working Party (RAWP) Report: sharing resources for health in England.* HMSO, London.
16 DHSS (1979) *Royal Commission on the NHS.* Cmnd 7615. HMSO, London.
17 DHSS (1979–80) *Clegg Commission on Pay Comparability.* HMSO, London.
18 DHSS (1979) *Patients First: consultative paper on the structure and management of the NHS in England and Wales.* HMSO, London.
19 DHSS (1980) *Black Report: inequalities in health. Report of a Research Working Group.* HMSO, London.
20 DHSS (1980) *Nodder Report: organisational and management problems of mental illness hospitals.* HMSO, London.
21 DHSS (1980) *Hospital Services: future pattern of hospital provision in England.* HMSO, London.
22 DHSS (1981) *Harding Report. The Primary Health Care Team: report of a Joint Working Group of the Standing Medical Advisory Committee and the Standing Nursing and Midwifery Advisory Committee.* Department of Health and Social Security, London.
23 DHSS (1982) *Körner Report. Report of the Steering Group on Health Services Information.* HMSO, London.
24 DHSS (1983) *Griffiths Report. NHS Management Inquiry Report.* Department of Health and Social Security, London.
25 DHSS (1983) *Ceri Davies Report. Under-used and surplus property in the NHS.* HMSO, London.

26 DHSS (1984) *Hart Report. The Report of the NHS Management Inquiry: implications for the organisation of the Department.* Department of Health and Social Security, London.

27 Ham C (1999) *Health Policy in Britain* (4e). Palgrave Publications Ltd, Basingstoke.

28 Harrison A and Dixon J (2000) *The NHS Facing the Future.* The King's Fund, London.

29 Interview with Sir Norman Fowler, London, July 2002.

30 Nelson SPU, 25/10. Volume 1.

31 Nelson SPU, 8/7. The decision to launch the Review appears to have been taken at a meeting between Thatcher and Fowler on 8 September 1982.

32 Nelson SPU, 95. Volume 1.

33 Turner G (1982) *The Daily Telegraph.* Articles appeared in the autumn of that year.

34 Thatcher M (1993) *The Downing Street Years.* Harper Collins, London.

35 Foot M (1973) *Aneurin Bevan: a biography, 1945–1960.* Davis-Poynter, London. There are many variations of this now famous comment.

36 Department of Health (1988) *Griffiths Report. Community Care: agenda for action.* Cmnd 849. HMSO, London.

37 *The Sun,* 2 February 1983.

38 Interview with Sir Kenneth Clarke, London, 18 April 2002.

39 Interview with Sir Graham Hart, London, August 2002.

40 Nelson SPU, 40/2. Volume 1.

41 Griffiths R (1991) *Seven Years of Progress: general management in the NHS.* Audit Commission Management Lecture No.3, 3 June 1991.

42 Nelson SPU, 40/9. Volume 6.

43 Nelson SPU, 40/2. Volume 2.

44 Nelson SPU, 40/1. Volume 1.

45 Nelson SPU, 40/2. Volume 3.

46 Hansard (1983) *Debate on the NHS.* 27 October. House of Commons, London.

47 Nelson 312, HSB.

48 Nelson HSB/0001/V0001–V00013.

49 Nelson HSB /0001/V0002, 19 March 1984.

50 Nelson SPU, 40/2. Volume 4.

51 Macpherson G (ed.) (1998) *From Administration to Management. Our NHS: a celebration of 50 years.* British Medical Association, London.

52 Enthoven A (1985) *Enthoven Report. Reflections on the Management of the NHS: an American looks at the incentives to efficiency in health services management in the UK.* Occasional Paper No. 5. Nuffield Provincial Hospitals Trust, London.

53 DHSS (1986) *Stanley Royd Inquiry. Report of a Committee of Inquiry into an Outbreak of Food Poisoning at the Stanley Royd Hospital.* Department of Health and Social Security, London.

54 Griffiths R (1986) *Community Care: an agenda for discussion.* Department of Health and Social Security, London.

55 Nelson 312/HSB. Health Service Supervisory Board, Second Meeting, 16 February 1984.

56 Nelson SPU, 40/9. Volume 1.

57 Personal correspondence with Victor Paige, October 2002, including access to his personal papers.

58 Nelson SPU, 40/9. Volume 4.

59 Nelson SPU, 40/9. Volume 2.

60 Nelson SPU, 40/9. Volume 7.

61 *The Sunday Times,* 25 November 1984.

62 Interview with Victor Paige, 26 February 2001.

63 Nelson SPU, 40/16. Volume 1.

64 Correspondence between Victor Paige and authors, 29 September 2003.

65 Nelson RFM. Volume 4.

66 Nelson SPU, 40/2. Volume 5.
67 Paige V (1985) *General Management in the NHS*. Address to Institute of Health Services Management Conference, Coventry, 11 June 1985.
68 Nelson HSB 0001/V0004.
69 Paige V (1986) Managing the managers. *Can Med Assoc Bull.* **134**: 64–8.
70 Nelson 360 MBW/9, NHS MB, 15 July 1985.
71 Nelson SPU 70.
72 Nelson EFS/34/2. Volume 1.
73 Nelson RFM1. Volume 4.
74 Nelson RFM1. Volume 5.
75 Nelson RFM1. Volume 8.
76 Nelson 302 FYU/33. Volume 1.
77 Nelson 302 FYU/33. Volume 2.
78 Nelson 360 MBW/0004.
79 Nelson 360 MBW/0008.
80 Nelson 360 MBW/0009.
81 Nelson 360 MBW/0010.
82 Interview with Sir Len Peach, Grantham, May 2002.
83 Draft of letter from Sir Peter Baldwin to Kenneth Stowe. Author's private papers, 15 April 1985.
84 Fowler N (1991) *Ministers Decide*. Chapmans, London.
85 Letter from Kenneth Clarke to Victor Paige, 11 June 1986. Private papers of Victor Paige.
86 Author's correspondence with Victor Paige, 17 September 2002.
87 Paige VG (1987) *The Development of General Management Within the NHS, with Particular Reference to the Role of the NHS Management Board*. Evidence of Victor Paige to Social Services Committee, April 1987. Author's private papers.
88 Efficiency Unit, Cabinet Office (1988) *Ibbs Report. Improving Management in Government: the next steps*. Efficiency Unit, Cabinet Office, London.
89 Paige V (1988) *A Memorandum on the Efficiency Unit's Treasury Report to the Prime Minister on the 'Next Steps'. The Treasury and Civil Service Committee.* Author's private papers.
90 DHSS (1986) *Cumberlege Report. Neighbourhood Nursing: a focus for care.* Department of Health and Social Security, London.
91 Interview with Sir Joe Pilling, London, February 2002.
92 DHSS (1987) *Hospital Medical Staffing. Achieving a Balance: plan for action.* Report issued on behalf of the UK Health Departments, the Joint Consultants Committee, and Chairmen of Regional Health Authorities. DHSS, London.
93 Department of Health (1988) *Acheson Report. Public Health in England: the Report of the Committee of Inquiry into the future development of the public health function.* Cmnd 289. HMSO, London.
94 Department of Health (1989) *Working for Patients: the Health Service caring for the 1990s.* HMSO, London.
95 Department of Health (1989) *A Strategy for Nursing, A Report of the Steering Committee, Department of Health, Nursing Division.* Department of Health, London.
96 Stowe K (1989) *On Caring for the National Health.* Nuffield Provincial Hospitals Trust, London.
97 Health Select Committee, 1986.
98 *NHS Management Bulletin*, Issue 3, no. 86. Department of Health, London.
99 Nelson HSB 0001/V00010.
100 Kingston W and Rowbottom R (1989) *Making General Management Work in the NHS*. Sigma Centre, Brunel University, Uxbridge.
101 Currie E (2002) *Diaries 1987–92*. Little & Brown, London.
102 Nelson 312/HSB/5. Volume 1.

103 Nelson HSB 0001/V00012.

104 Nelson 360 MBW 48/53/54 302 FYU 33 volume 2, 3 BHX V0001-5.

105 Department of Health (2000) *Shaping the Future NHS: long-term planning for hospitals and related services*. Department of Health, London.

106 Meeting between RHA Chairmen and Ministers. Author's private diary, 18 November 1997.

107 Campbell J (2003) *Margaret Thatcher. Volume 2. The Iron Lady*. Cape, London, p. 509.

108 Rivett G (1998) *From Cradle to Grave. Fifty years of the NHS*. The King's Fund, London.

109 Edwards B (1995) *The National Health Service: a manager's tale. 1946–1994*. Nuffield Provincial Hospitals Trust, London.

110 Author's private diary, submission by regional health authority chairmen and regional general managers to the 1988 health service review, dated 14 March 1988.

111 Timmins N (2001) *The Five Giants. A Biography of the Welfare State*. Harper Collins, London.

112 Nelson 360 MBW/54, 5 October 1987.

113 *The Times*, 8 April 1989.

114 Regional chairs' meeting, November 1987. Author's private diary.

115 Letter to regional chairs from Tony Newton about the financial position, 23 December 1987. Author's private papers.

116 *The Independent*, 7 December 1987.

117 Klein R (2001) *The New Politics of the NHS* (4e). Prentice Hall, Harlow.

118 Lawson N (1992) *The View from No 11*. Bantam, London.

119 Nelson 312 HSB/9.

120 Interview with Sir Christopher France, January 2002.

121 Major J (1999) *The Autobiography*. Harper Collins, London.

122 Review will protect right to free health care, says Moore. *The Times*, 26 April 1988.

123 Split over tax incentives to boost private health cover. *The Times*, 8 June 1988.

124 Nelson NHS MB BHX V0001 1/8/88, NHS MB paper [88]8.

125 Correspondence between Kenneth Clarke and authors, 22 September 2003.

126 Nurses demand more cash for 'oxygen starved' NHS. *The Times*, 25 May 1988.

127 Life and death on the NHS: cost and the future of the NHS. *The Times*, 23 May 1988.

128 Nelson, NHS MB Meeting 3/10/88 BHX V0015.

129 Response of Chris France to Donald Wilson. *Responsibilities and Structure of the DHSS*, 29 March 1988. Author's private papers.

130 Timmins N (1989) Is the NHS safe in their hands? *The Independent*, 9 February.

131 Department of Health (1989) *Working for Patients: implications for Family Practitioner Committees*. Working Paper 8 (includes key changes for Family Practitioner Services). Department of Health, London.

132 IHSM (1989) *Reviewing the Review*. Institute of Health Services Management, London.

133 National Association of Health Authorities briefing, 15 February 1989.

134 Owen D (1989) Unhealthy prescription for the NHS. *The Daily Telegraph*, 31 January.

135 Hennessey P (1989) *Caring for People: community care in the next decade and beyond*. HMSO, London.

136 Department of Health (1991) *Junior Doctors: the new deal. Calman Report*. HMSO, London.

137 Department of Health (1991) *The Patient's Charter*. HMSO, London.

138 Department of Health (1991) *Health of the Nation*. HMSO, London.

139 Department of Health (1992) *Tomlinson Report. Report of the Inquiry into London's Health Service, Medical Education and Research*. HMSO, London.

140 Department of Health (1994) *Managing the New NHS. Functions and Responsibilities in the New NHS (Jenkins Review)*. Department of Health, London.

141 Department of Health (1994) *Clothier Report (Allitt Inquiry). Independent Inquiry Relating*

to Deaths and Injuries on the Children's Ward at Grantham and Kesteven General Hospital during February to April 1991. HMSO, London.

142 Department of Health (1994) *Banks Report. Review of the Wider Department of Health.* Department of Health, London.

143 Department of Health (1989) *Working for Patients.* HMSO, London.

144 Nelson 477 VKC. Volume 1.

145 NHS Policy Board, 30 September 1992. Paper PB [92] 37. Author's private papers.

146 Briefing for the Public Accounts Committee hearing, 16 February 1994. Author's private papers.

147 Interview with Sir Duncan Nichol, Manchester, 14 August 2001.

148 Department of Health Circular EL(89)MB 102, May 1990.

149 *The Times,* 5 April 1989.

150 Nichol D (1989) Working for Patients. The role of managers in implementing the White Paper. *Health Services Management.* **85**(3).

151 Nelson NHS MB, November 1990.

152 Countdown to April 1991. Comment. *Health Serv J.* 14 June 1990.

153 Nichol D (1995) The managerial revolution: medicine as a business. *Med Educ.* **29 (Suppl.1):** 41–3.

154 NHS PB, 28 November 1989. Author's private papers.

155 Letter from Duncan Nichol to Sir Anthony Grabham, 22 September 1989. Author's private papers.

156 Department of Health (1990) *Briefing for Managers [3. 44].* Department of Health, London.

157 Crail M (1996) Behind the scenes at the NHS. *Health Serv J.*

158 Department of Health (1989) *Briefing for NHS Managers. Self-governing Hospitals.* Department of Health, London.

159 Parliamentary Question, 20 February 1990.

160 Moore W and Sheldon T (1990) Department of Health set to put brakes on pace of reform. *Health Serv J.* 29 March 1990.

161 East Anglian Regional Health Authority (1990) *Rubber Windmill 1. Market Simulation Exercise.* East Anglian Regional Health Authority, Cambridge.

162 Department of Health (1990) Press release 90/324. Department of Health, London.

163 NHS Policy Board (1990) Author's private papers, 26 September.

164 NHS Policy Board (1990) Author's private papers, 31 October.

165 Department of Health (1989) Letter to RGMs, 14 March 1989. Author's private papers.

166 Letter from Kenneth Clarke to all MPs, 18 June 1990.

167 Interview with Virginia Bottomley, London, September 2001.

168 *Management Systems and Planning Guidance for 1991–92.* Circular. EL[90]207, 24 October 1990. Department of Health, London.

169 DHA Project Newsletter. Issue 2, August 1990. Department of Health, London.

170 Ham C (1992) *Holding On, Letting Go. A Report on the Relationship Between Directly Managed Units and District Health Authorities.* The King's Fund, London.

171 William Waldegrave speaking on the television programme, *The Right Prescription,* broadcast on BBC2 in 1990.

172 Circular EL [90] 218, 20 November 1990. Department of Health, London.

173 NHS Policy Board, 28 November 1990. Author's private papers.

174 William Waldegrave speaking at the Annual Conservative Central Council meeting, Southport, on 23 March 1991.

175 NHS Policy Board, 28 November 1990. Author's private diary.

176 Department of Health (1991) *Joint Guidance for Hospital Consultants on GP Fundholding.* Press release H91/255 and EL [91]84. Department of Health, London.

177 Presentation to the Prime Minister by Duncan Nichol and Sheila Masters. Briefing note, 15 July 1991. Author's private papers.

178 NHS Policy Board (1991) *The Communication Programme.* PB[91]10. Author's private papers.

179 Nelson BHM/0009/V0005 Policy Board and author's private papers, 30 October 1991.

180 NHS Management Executive (1992) *Annual Report, 1991–92.* NHS Management Executive, Leeds.

181 Interview with William Waldegrave, London, November 2001 and meeting between Secretary of State and Regional Chairs on 16 January 1991.

182 *The Wilson Letter,* March 1991. Author's private diary and papers.

183 Public Accounts Committee (1994) *Advances to Health Authorities in England 1992–93.* HMSO, London.

184 *Daily Mail,* October 1991 and letter from D Nichol in *Health Serv J.* 17 November 1991.

185 NHS puts Major on the defensive. *The Times,* 8 October 1991.

186 Leathley A (1991) Health Chief accused by Union. *The Times,* 8 October 1991.

187 Dented shield. *Health Serv J.* 10 October 1991.

188 Public Accounts Committee (1993) *West Midlands Regional Health Authority: regionally managed services organisation.* Press notice on 57th PAC Report. Public Accounts Committee, House of Commons, London.

189 *The Bromsgrove Experiment, 1990–1997 and Beyond.* University of Birmingham, Birmingham.

190 Secretary of State for Health (1998) *The Health of the Nation: a policy assessed.* The Stationery Office, London.

191 Interview with Frank Dobson, London, November 2002.

192 NHS Policy Board, 27 June 1990. Paper PB [90] 12. Author's private papers.

193 Nick Ross. Interview with Virginia Bottomley on the BBC television programme *On the Record,* broadcast on 12 February 1993.

194 NHS Policy Board (1989) PB 89 annex A. Author's private papers.

195 Nelson 477 VKB/0001 /0008, 477 VKB/0001/0009, BHM9 Volume 5, BHM12 Volume 4.

196 NHS Policy Board, 30 September 1992. Paper PB [92] 37. Author's private papers.

197 Department of Health (1992) Press release H92/142. Department of Health, London.

198 Letter to Board members, 23 October 1992. Author's private papers.

199 *Messages and reactions,* 20 October 1993, a briefing note prepared at the launch of *Managing the New NHS.* Author's private papers.

200 Warden J (1998) Role of the CMO is eroded. *BMJ.* **317:** 1340.

201 Hunt J (1994) Hospitals two-tier waiting-list shock. *Birmingham Mail,* 14 February.

202 Langlands' speech to the NAHAT/IHSM conference, *Managing the New NHS,* 24 January 1994. This paper was widely circulated by Langlands' team.

203 Department of Health (1994) *Managing the New NHS: a background document.* Department of Health, London.

204 NHS Executive (1994) *The Operation of the NHS Internal Market: local freedoms, national responsibilities.* Department of Health, London.

205 Department of Health and the Welsh Office (1995) *A Policy Framework for Commissioning Cancer Services (Calman–Hine Report).* Department of Health and Welsh Office, London and Cardiff.

206 (1995) *Challenges and Policy Options. Healthcare 2000 Report: UK health and health services.* Chaired by Duncan Nichol and funded by the Pharmaceutical Industry. Health 2000. Shirehall Communications, London. See also Crail M and Butler P (2005) What's on Sir Duncan's agenda? *Health Serv J.* 9 February.

207 Webster C (1996) *The Health Services Since the War. Volume 2.* The Stationery Office, London.

208 Department of Health (1996) *The National Health Service: a service with ambitions.* HMSO, London.

209 Department of Health (1997) *The New NHS: modern, dependable.* The Stationery Office, London.
210 Department of Health (1999) *Report of the Inquiry into the Personality Disorder Unit, Ashworth Special Hospital (Fallon Inquiry).* Cmnd 4194-1. The Stationery Office, London.
211 Department of Health (1998) *Our Healthier Nation: a contract for health.* The Stationery Office, London.
212 Department of Health (1998) *A First-Class Service: quality in the new NHS.* The Stationery Office, London.
213 (1998) Dobson announces beds inquiry. *BMJ.* **317** (10 October).
214 Department of Health (1998) *Independent Inquiry into Inequalities in Health (Acheson Report).* The Stationery Office, London.
215 Department of Health (2001) *Your Guide to the NHS.* The Stationery Office, London.
216 Interview with Alan Langlands, Dundee, September 2002.
217 Watts G (1999) Crisis. What crisis. *BMJ.* **318:** 270.
218 Interview with Ken Jarrold, Durham, December 2001.
219 NHS Management Executive, 21 March 1994. Author's private papers.
220 Department of Health (1995) *Statement of Responsibilities and Accountabilities.* Department of Health, London.
221 Crail M (1995) All above board. *Health Serv J.* 9 March.
222 Pritchard W (1994) *Board Effectiveness.* Report by external consultant. Author's private papers.
223 Hunter H (1995) Calculated snub. Report of Discussion Paper 134. *Health Serv J.* 8 June.
224 As Langlands pointed out in his lecture to the World Productivity Conference in Edinburgh in October 1999, you have to add the contribution of the private health sector of 0.9% to get a true comparator of roughly 6.8%, compared with an average European figure at that time of more than 8%.
225 (1996) Another year older and deeper in debt. *Health Serv J.* 12 December.
226 Butler P (1995) Road to full local bargaining is rocky one. *Health Serv J.* 12 January.
227 Butler P (1995) Trust moot massive pay shake-up. *Health Serv J.* 20 April.
228 Butler P (1995) RCN hints at agreement on local pay. *Health Serv J.* 4 May.
229 Department of Health (1995) *Almost 90% of Trusts Have Made Offers to Their Nursing Staff.* Press release 95/332. Department of Health, London.
230 Snell J (1995) Jarrold urges trusts to make local pay deals to head off strike action. *Health Serv J.* 27 July.
231 Butler P (1995) Paying up. *Health Serv J.* 20 July.
232 Abberley R (1996) Address to National Association of Health Authorities and Trusts conference. *Health Serv J.* 19 September.
233 NHS Policy Board, October 1995. Author's private papers.
234 Crail M (1995) Keeping the peace. *Health Serv J.* 14 September.
235 Hancock C (1995) Is local pay worth the trouble? *Health Serv J.* 6 July.
236 Department of Health (1995) *Gerald Malone Welcomes Continued Expansion of GP Fundholding.* Press release 95/254. Department of Health, London.
237 Langlands A (1995) Secrecy in the NHS. Letter to the *British Medical Journal* in response to letter by Craft and others that appeared on 17 December 1994 under the heading 'The rise of Stalinism in the NHS'. *BMJ* (1994) **309:** 1640–5.
238 Crail M (1995) Most trust managers claim NHS secrecy has increased. *Health Serv J.* 2 February.
239 Davies P (1995) A vision beyond winners and losers. *Health Serv J.* 2 February.
240 Merkel K (1995) How the 'Woman of integrity and courage' has let us all down. *Health Serv J.* 13 April.

241 Cervi B (1995) Department of Health vetoes hit list for rationing. *Health Serv J.* 2 November.

242 Chadda D (1996) Dorrell condemns blanket ban on treatments. *Health Serv J.* 11 January.

243 Chadda D (1995) Child B health commission would fund evaluated care. *Health Serv J.* 24 August.

244 Profile. The girl who conquered cancer – and the NHS. *The Sunday Times*, 29 October 1995.

245 Rational planning (editorial). *The Times*, 27 October 1995.

246 Crail M (1995) The facts of life. *Health Serv J.* 9 November.

247 (1995) *Health Serv J.* 2 March.

248 National Audit Office (1996) *Inquiry Commissioned by the NHS Chief Executive into Matters Concerning the Former Yorkshire RHA. Report by the Comptroller and Auditor General.* HMSO, London.

249 Butler P (1996) Tales of muck and brass. *Health Serv J.* 21 March.

250 Butler P (1996) *The Fall Guy?* McLean Interview. *Health Serv J.* 20 June.

251 Langlands A (1996) Promoting 'The Health of the Nation'. A–Z of management and finance in the NHS. *Br J Hosp Med.* **56**: 171–2.

252 Murray I (1998) Curb on Caesarean births to save costs. *The Times*, 6 March.

253 (1995) The end is nigh for Mrs Bottomley. *Health Serv J.* 13 April.

254 (1995) Will history repeat itself? *Health Serv J.* 13 July.

255 Interview with Alan Milburn, London, 21 January 2004.

256 NHS Executive (1995) *Briefing for New Ministers.* Author's private papers.

257 Interview with Stephen Dorrell, 12 December 2001.

258 *The Times*, 10 December 1997.

259 Crail M (1995) Danger money. *Health Serv J.* 1 June.

260 (1995) Now it's the battle to win the peace. *Health Serv J.* 3 August.

261 (1995) Manager bashing is an easy option. *Health Serv J.* 24 August.

262 (1996) A bunch of fives from Mr Dorrell. *Health Serv J.* 9 May.

263 (1996) Caines attacks Dorrell's 'slurs' on managers. *Health Serv J.* 11 July.

264 NHS Executive (1996) *Seeing the Wood, Sparing the Trees.* Department of Health, London.

265 Chadda D and Cervi B (1996) Managers will not lose jobs. *Health Serv J.* 3 October.

266 (1996) Poor performing trusts could be closed down. Conference focus. *Health Serv J.* 9 September.

267 *The Times*, 29 October 1994.

268 (1996) Dorrell furious at Roger's handling of Read codes row. *Health Serv J.* 27 June.

269 Cross M (1998) Langlands blames Nichol for Read codes fiasco. *Health Serv J.* 26 March.

270 Lilley R (2000) The Complete Roy Lilley Guide. *Health Serv J.* 9 March.

271 Department of Health (1996) *Primary Care: delivering the future.* Department of Health, London.

272 Adapted from analysis in *Health Service Journal* (10 April 1997), *The Sunday Times* (13 May 2001) and *The Times* (21 June 2001).

273 (1997) News Focus. *Health Serv J.* 18 December.

274 *The Times*, 1997.

275 Telephone interview with Frank Dobson and Brian Edwards, 28 September 2003.

276 (1998) *Health Serv J.* 19 February.

277 Turnberg Report on London, February 1998. Department of Health, London.

278 At the Labour Party Conference in Blackpool in 1998 Dobson announced a Beds Inquiry, which reported in 2000.

279 (1998) *BMJ.* **317** (16 July).

280 Crisp N (2002) *Chief Executive's Report to NHS.* Department of Health, London.

281 Edwards B (ed.) (1999) *Shaping the NHS. NHS Fiftieth Anniversary lectures.* NHS Executive, Leeds.

282 (2000) Milburn defends PFI at Select Committee. *BMJ.* **321:** 1025.

283 Butler P (1999) Suits you, Sir. *Health Serv J.* 1 April.

284 (1999) *With Respect to Old Age: long-term care – rights and responsibilities. A report by the Royal Commission on Long-Term Care.* Cmnd 4192-1. The Stationery Office, London.

285 Department of Health (1999) *Saving Lives: our healthier nation.* The Stationery Office, London.

286 Appelby J (1999) *Health Serv J.* March.

287 Ferriman A (1998) Doctors ration treatment for heart patients. *The Independent,* 21 June.

288 Klein R (1998) A generous birthday present for the NHS. *BMJ.* **317:** 224.

289 Dargie C (2000) *Policy Futures for UK Health. 2000 Report.* The Stationery Office, London.

290 Sherman J (1999) Milburn tells NHS to speed up reform. *The Times,* 14 October.

291 Department of Health (1999) *Modernisation Here to Stay.* Press release 1999/0611. Department of Health, London.

292 Alan Langlands' statement to the Bristol Royal Infirmary Inquiry in March 2002. Author's private papers.

293 *New Statesman,* January 2000.

294 (2000) GDP spend dubbed cynical. *Health Serv J.* 20 January.

295 Sherman J (2000) NHS Chief quits for a new life at university. *The Times,* 22 February.

296 Sherman J (2000) Doctors and nurses drafted in to manage NHS. *The Times,* 23 February.

297 Dean M (2000) A new NHS revolution causes trouble. *Lancet.* 4 March.

298 (1995) Leadership. *Health Serv J.* 24 August.

299 Sherman J (2000) How Blair came late to reform of the NHS. *The Times,* 23 April.

300 Department of Health (2000) *Milburn Insists Front-Line NHS Services Must Benefit from New Money.* Press release 2000/0183. Department of Health, London.

301 Baldwin T and Wright O (2003) Hospital waiting list figures 'are being distorted'. *The Times,* 4 March.

302 Department of Health (2000) *New Post at the Top of the Department of Health.* Press release 2000/0338. Department of Health, London.

303 Charter D (2001) Ministers try to head off NHS mutiny. *The Times,* 23 April.

304 McGauran A and Donnelly L (2000) Making plans for Nigel. *Health Serv J.* 19 October.

305 Department of Health (2001) *Milburn Hands Power to Front-Line Staff.* Press release 2001/0200. Department of Health, London.

306 Crisp N (2001) Department of Health Special Bulletin Number 7.

307 Gould M (2001) Election focus. *Health Serv J.* 3 May.

308 (2001) Scant regard for job fears. *Health Serv J.* 3 May.

309 Timmins N (2001) Spin-doctors are killing the health service. *Financial Times,* 16 July.

310 Prime Minister's speech on reform of the public services at the Royal Free Hospital London. Downing Street news-room, 16 July 2001.

311 Conservatives are committed to a free NHS. *The Times,* 11 May 2001.

312 Lib Dems seek dedicated tax to fund the NHS. *The Times,* 16 July 2001.

313 (2001) News. *BMJ* (8 December).

314 Crisp N (2001) *Focusing on Delivery.* Department of Health, London.

315 (2003) NHS and social care interest. *Chief Executive's Bulletin,* Issue 153. Department of Health, London.

316 (1998) Milburn agreed that Merit award would not be for life but must be earned. *BMJ* (15 June).

317 Department of Health (1999) *Major Reduction in NHS Fraud.* Press release 1999/0787. Department of Health, London.

318 (2001) *BMJ*. **322** (9 June).

319 Moore W (2000) *Wanless Report Sparks Debate on Funding of Health Service*. See also Ferriman A (2001) Blair backlash on European average. *BMJ*. **323**: 1325.

320 Bogle I (2001) Opening address to BMA Conference, 2001. *BMJ*. **323** (7 July).

321 Consultants ready to quit NHS. *The Times*, 6 March 2003.

322 Milburn's speech to the NHS Confederation Conference, 6 July 2001.

323 Department of Health (2001) *Health Reforms Need Public Service Ethos*. Press release 2001/0309. Department of Health, London.

324 Prime Minister's speech on public service reform. Downing Street news-room, 16 October 2001.

325 The Treasury (2001) *Wanless Report: interim report on NHS funding*; www.hm-treasury.gov.uk

326 Smith D (2001) So how do you want to pay for it? *The Sunday Times*, 2 December.

327 (2001) Obituary for the NHS. *The Sunday Times*, 11 November.

328 Webster P and Paterson L (2001) Brown will raise taxes to revive the NHS. *The Times*, 28 November.

329 (2001) Minister will order NHS to shift power to local hospitals. *The Times*, 2 December.

330 Charter D (2003) Belgium to take on 1000 NHS patients. *The Times*, 8 February.

331 *Redefining the NHS*. Milburn's speech to the New Health Network, 15 January 2002.

332 *The Times*, 7 February 2002.

333 Charter D (2002) Milburn 'takes NHS beyond Thatcherism'. *The Times*, 7 May.

334 Department of Health (2002) *Delivering the NHS Plan: next steps*. The Stationery Office, London.

335 Letter from Downing Street to NHS Chief Executives, 18 April 2002. Author's private papers.

336 Hospital reformers revive Brown/Milburn clash. *The Times*, 1 March 2003.

337 Buckley C (2003) End of healthcare as we know it. *The Times*, 15 July.

338 *Localism: from rhetoric to reality*. Secretary of State's speech to the New Health Network and New Local Government Network, 5 February 2003.

339 Hawkes N (2002) New GP trusts could inherit debts of £1.5 billion. *The Times*, 1 April.

340 *BMJ*. **324** (30 March).

341 *BMJ*. **324** (20 April).

342 *Chief Executive's Bulletin*, 7–14 March 2003. Department of Health, London.

343 Dyson R (2003) *Why the New NHS Will Fail, and What Should Replace It*. Matthew James Publishing Ltd, Chelmsford.

344 Department of Health; www.doh.gov.uk

345 Department of Health (2003) *Why We Are Changing*. Department of Health, London.

346 Wanless D (2004) *Securing Good Health for the Whole Population*. Department of Health, London.

347 Interview with David Hinchliffe MP, Wakefield, June 2002.

348 McConnel H (2001) *Lost Bedpans*. Political Economy Research Centre, University of Sheffield, Sheffield.

349 Cooper C (1995) Separating policy from operations in the Prison Service. A case study. *Public Policy Admin J*. **10**: 4.

350 For a thorough analysis of accountability see Woods K (2002) *A Critical Appraisal of Accountability Structures in Integrated Health Systems*. Scottish Executive, Edinburgh.

351 Department of Health (2003) *NHS and Social Care Bulletin*. Department of Health, London.

352 *Medicine's Missing Millions*, broadcast on BBC television programme *Panorama* on 6 January 1997.

353 Palmer J (2003) Doctors' leader blasts Labour target. *Daily Mirror*, 1 July.

354 Moore A (2002) When Nanny got in a state. *Health Serv J*. 20 June.

355 Brindle D (1998) Chief to quit NHS if fees imposed. *Guardian*, 4 July.

356 Crisp N (2003) Diagnosing the ailments of the NHS (letter). *The Times*, 6 October.

357 Enthoven A (2002) *Future of the NHS. Rock Carling Lecture*. Nuffield Trust, London.

358 Department of Health (2003) *Government Departments Must Lead Efficiency by Example, Reid Tells Select Committee*. Press release 2003/0417. Department of Health, London.

359 Wooding D (2002) Don't blame us, guv. *The Sun*, 2 February.

360 King's Fund (2002) *The Future of the NHS*. King's Fund, London.

361 Department of Health (1995) *Changes to the NHS Policy Board*. Press release 95/512. Department of Health, London.

362 Bottomley V (1995) Lecture delivered to the Royal Society of Medicine, 20 June 1995. Author's private papers.

363 Health Financial Management Association (2004–05) *NHS Finance in the UK* (7e). HFMA, Bristol.

364 The NHS and Community Care Bill 1990.

365 Report by Sir Christopher France, Policy Board No. 7, 28 February 1990. Author's private papers.

366 Dyke G (1998) *The New NHS Charter: a different approach*. Department of Health, London.

367 World Health Organization (1978) *Alma Ata. WHO Conference on Primary Health Care*. WHO, Geneva.

368 Wright O (2003) Milburn attacks central control. *The Times*, 6 March.

369 Robertson D and Carr-Brown J (2003) Private firms to run family doctor services. *The Times*, 21 December.

370 Hawkes N (2004) Doctors want all patients to buy insurance. *The Times*, 25 February.

371 Timmins N (2004) Pledge to halt culture of targets. *The Financial Times*, 18 March.

372 Timmins N (2004) Health service gets more business-like. *The Financial Times*, 16 June.

373 *Health for All in the Year 2000*. World Health Organization, Geneva.

374 Carr-Brown J (2002) NHS 'big bang' will give GPs new powers. *The Sunday Times*, 31 March.

375 NHS Executive Meeting, January 1996. Author's private paper.

376 NHS Executive Board Meeting, April 1995. Author's private paper.

377 Hunt P (2004) Foundation freedoms. *Health Serv J*. 11 November.

378 Department of Health (2000) *The NHS Plan: a plan for investment, a plan for reform*. Cmnd 4818-1. DoH, London.

379 Department of Health Press Release 2000/0752.

380 Department of Health (2001) *Reforming the Mental Health Act*. Cmnd 5016-1. DoH, London.

381 *Shifting the Balance of Power in the NHS*. Speech by Alan Milburn, 25 April 2001.

Index